'This book is a rare and invaluable contribution to the field of therapeutic work with children. The writers bring both deep compassion and clinical clarity to the delivery and impact of play based occupational therapy. With rich case studies and grounded theory, this book bridges the gap between evidence-based practice and the lived realities of working with children who carry complex trauma'.

'The authors manage to articulate what many clinicians feel but struggle to express: that within the simplicity of play lies extraordinary potential for healing, connection, and transformation. A must-read for all professionals committed to supporting the most vulnerable young people, with skill, sensitivity and heart'.

Rhona McAlpine, *specialist occupational therapist, parent infant therapist*

'A practical and thoughtful guide, bridging theory and clinical practice. Drawing on their expertise as seasoned clinicians, the authors seamlessly integrate case studies that provide profound insights, reflections, and practical wisdom. This resource equips professionals with an essential understanding when using play based approaches to support children and young people who have experienced complex trauma. A must read!'

Sara Shafi, *PhD, consultant clinical psychologist, Specialist Trauma Team, NHS Lothian*

'How can services best meet the needs of children and young people with complex trauma? This clear and accessible book is invaluable for anyone working in Children's Services and CAMHS. It is a testimony to the importance of understanding children's ways of communicating through play and the centrality of relationship-based practice as well as the challenges involved in this way of working'.

Debbie Hindle, *PhD, child and adolescent psychotherapist, Human Development Scotland*

CHILD-LED THERAPY FOR CHILDREN WITH COMPLEX TRAUMA

Taking an occupational therapy perspective, this book provides a resource for practitioners from many disciplines working with children who have experienced complex trauma. Readers are reminded of the damage done to these children and the challenges faced by professionals when communicating with them. Play is one way in, and the overriding message is that children's play needs to be taken very seriously both for healthy development and as a therapeutic medium to support children's wellbeing.

Written in accessible language and supported throughout by examples of children's play and artwork, chapters provide a bedrock of well-explained theory with links to practice. Topics explored include:

- Recognising and understanding complex trauma
- Using play as a means of communication
- Child-led assessment and play based occupational therapy
- Exploration about what happens in the therapy room
- Occupational therapists as part of the multidisciplinary team
- The necessary support structures for therapists

An essential text for any therapist working in the field of children's mental health, this book provides readers with an effective approach in their clinical work with children and their families, bringing together an understanding of trauma, psychodynamic theory and play.

Gita Ingram is an occupational therapist and systemic practitioner who worked in a child and adolescent mental health service as Head of Occupational Therapy and then manager of a specialist team for children in the care system. She is now an independent trainer and consultant, and writes about play and psychodynamic approaches.

Susie Reade is an occupational therapist who worked in a child and adolescent mental health service as clinical specialist in the sexual trauma team. She is now learning British Sign Language and volunteering in services for deaf children. She is an exhibiting visual artist.

Annie Green is an occupational therapist and counsellor who worked for many years in a child and adolescent mental health service as head of occupational therapy and clinical specialist in the child trauma team. She is now an exhibiting visual artist.

CHILD-LED THERAPY FOR CHILDREN WITH COMPLEX TRAUMA

Just Playing?

Gita Ingram, Susie Reade and Annie Green

Routledge
Taylor & Francis Group

LONDON AND NEW YORK

Designed cover image: Gita Ingram, Susie Reade and Annie Green

First published 2026
by Routledge
4 Park Square, Milton Park, Abingdon, Oxon OX14 4RN

and by Routledge
605 Third Avenue, New York, NY 10158

Routledge is an imprint of the Taylor & Francis Group, an informa business

For Product Safety Concerns and Information please contact our EU representative GPSR@taylorandfrancis.com. Taylor & Francis Verlag GmbH, Kaufingerstraße 24, 80331 München, Germany.

British Library Cataloguing-in-Publication Data
A catalogue record for this book is available from the British Library

ISBN: 9781041079248 (hbk)
ISBN: 9781041079224 (pbk)
ISBN: 9781003642862 (ebk)

DOI: 10.4324/9781003642862

Typeset in Joanna
by codeMantra

CONTENTS

Foreword   ix
Preface   xii
Acknowledgements   xvi

Introduction and chapter outlines   1

1   Understanding complex trauma   10

2   Additional vulnerabilities to trauma   22

3   Play as communication and as a child's natural occupation   32

4   What happens in the playroom   41

5   Assessment, review and planning   58

6   Theoretical underpinning of play based occupational therapy   74

7   The therapeutic process   93

8   Working with the multidisciplinary team   110

9   Supervision and support   124

     Final thoughts   132

     Index   135

FOREWORD

From the onset of my career in occupational therapy, I was preoccupied with the idea of becoming a therapist and what that meant in relation to my developing understanding of using meaningful activities/occupations to improve wellbeing. The focus upon meaning was always the crux but I discovered that 'therapy' was an elastic concept and that therapists came in many different types. Also, perhaps more attention was paid both in professional education and practice to acquiring the unique skill set rather than to understanding the attendant therapeutic process. It was fortunate indeed, if a student placement or a work setting included being supervised by a person who had regard for and instilled the ideas of how to listen, make sense of behaviour and unravel meaning, learn to turn-take and fully engage and be 'present' with another person or group. Those foundations of therapeutic engagement and the therapeutic process are aspects which require continual reflection and refinement throughout practice and our careers. Indeed, those skills and attributes based upon critical reflexivity and constant exploration of process are invaluable in areas such as leadership, education and research.

This book offers a masterclass in understanding how to carefully explore the meaning of becoming a therapist and through words and pictures reveals insight into dealing with complex trauma. It engages the reader and stresses respectfulness, humility and empathy within therapeutic exchanges. Equally attention is paid to how the therapist requires to access personal supervision to remain in touch with their own learning, become aware of blind spots in their thinking and nurture development of understanding and skill. High levels of sensitivity to the way in which children and young people sought to communicate their hurt and distress are evident in every chapter and the intensity of each encounter is portrayed. It is explained that traumatised children can become traumatised adults and that the value of child-led therapy at an early stage in life can provide the aspect of strengthening a sense of self and activating the other keystone of therapy which is to exploring resilience strategies. Resilience and ways to promote positive change in children are revealed in the way they use the play space and begin to put words to feelings. This important emotional progress is most vividly shown within the Introduction and Carrie's entry to therapy and then again within the final vignette of Carrie (Final thoughts) when she proclaims, 'it's just as well I've learned how to drive'.

All chapters deal with complexity, subtlety and nuanced emotional puzzles whether dealing with theory or the components of the therapeutic process. As stated within the text, there are different reasons that a child or young person might be referred to CAMHS for help with complex trauma but that one of the underlying messages for the therapist is 'how to think about the unthinkable'. This is an invitation to go beyond the immediate and presenting issues and seek to provide a safe space both physically and emotionally to jointly explore.

The title conveys this invitation from the onset in the juxtaposition of the words in the title of 'complex trauma' and implicit question of 'just playing?' This is a text which represents the combined extensive and unique expertise of three therapists, who over the years have constantly honed their therapeutic skills and worked with children and young people who have experienced psychological and physical trauma. As is outlined in Chapter 1, the dictionary definition of 'trauma' means the effect or consequences of a wound or to pierce, and in this book, there is a rich description from both words and pictures of the effects upon children and young people of being wounded and trying to find ways that this can be communicated and subsequently managed. That is the essence of therapy in this setting.

The Scottish Government have stated that the current target of referral to a CAMHS unit is within 18 weeks and that this was met towards the end of

2024. A positive emphasis is placed upon the budgetary resources allocated to community and school-based interventions and that those referred to CAMHS represent a small number. It would be heartening to think that those intended preventative measures are improving the life chances and experience for troubled children and young people. However, the examples given in Chapters 1 and 2 of types of complex trauma and the reasons for referral have not diminished but arguably are escalating within present society. I would therefore endorse the strong messages in this book of recognising the impact of complex trauma, the need for early intervention, interdisciplinary and interagency support, and especially for retaining child-led play based therapy.

As stated by Nelson Mandela, humanitarian and former president of South Africa 'there can be no keener revelation of a society's soul than the way in which it treats its children' (Address at the launch of the Nelson Mandela Children's Fund, Pretoria 1995).

Dr. Sheena E. E. Blair Dip COT, M Ed, Ed D, FCOT

PREFACE

As a small group of occupational therapists working in a Child and Adolescent Mental Health Service (CAMHS), we all shared a thirst for finding a fit for psychoanalytic concepts within occupational therapy. The idea that play is a child's natural occupation and a powerful therapeutic medium was familiar to us when we started practising. The term non-directive play was often used. How could this be further developed by an enhanced understanding of the role of the unconscious in communication with children, and indeed their families and the organisations around them?

This development seemed particularly urgent as the understanding of the effects of complex trauma grew and brought together two disciplines once distinctly apart, those of neuropsychology and psychoanalysis. In addition, increased knowledge of child development and attachment processes dovetailed with those disciplines. We understood that, for us, non-directive therapy alone is not sufficient to help children process and recover from trauma and that child-led play was a more accurate term to describe trauma-informed therapy. It is helpful for the child to know that the therapist is informed of and can hold in mind what has happened to them, whilst being in tune with how they choose to communicate in the session. At the heart of our endeavours was a drive to maintain the role of play as central in clinical practice in CAMHS, regardless of professional background.

Psychoanalysis has much to offer many professional groups outside of psychotherapy itself. Psychoanalytic theory underpinned our occupational therapy practice. We found that the development opportunities offered by Human Development Scotland, previously known as The Scottish Institute of Human Relations (SIHR), provided a lifeline for us professionally. We each have completed all or part of the course 'Psychoanalytic Observation and Reflective Practice: Therapeutic Skills for Children and Young People'. This training also gave us a peer group of likeminded colleagues of many professional backgrounds including occupational therapy.

This was the backdrop to our great excitement when we found ourselves at the Masterclass on Psychoanalytic Thinking in Occupational Therapy at Brunel University in 2013, organised by Dr. Lindsay Nicholls and Italian occupational therapists and creators of the Vivaio model of occupational therapy (MOVI), Carolina de Sena Gibertoni and Julie Cunningham Piergrossi. These were inspirational days! We are grateful to them and to Dr. Sheena Blair who contributed to the conferences so wholeheartedly. They, alongside Margaret Daniel, published *Psychoanalytic Thinking in Occupational Therapy* (2013). We in Edinburgh continued to meet to share our work, to exchange ideas and to dream of the book we would one day write, describing our model as play based occupational therapy.

The three of us who have brought this book into fruition are indebted to our CAMHS occupational therapy colleagues Heather Hunter, Lorna Pearson and Jette Lemvig who over the years enriched our writing group and provided practical ideas and thoughtful reflection about the case material in this publication. Dr. Heather Hunter became Senior Lecturer in Occupational Therapy at Queen Margaret University, Edinburgh, promoting in particular the MOVI psychoanalytically based occupational therapy model. Sadly, Heather died in 2024. We miss her greatly. Lorna Pearson continues to practice in CAMHS where she further develops play based occupational therapy. Jette Lemvig has moved on to working as an occupational therapist in the field of adoption and fostering.

Thank you also to our peer reviewers: Sheena Blair, Debbie Hindle, Sara Shafi and Molly Ludlam, whose anonymised reviews at the start of our journey with Routledge publishers, provided us with such encouragement.

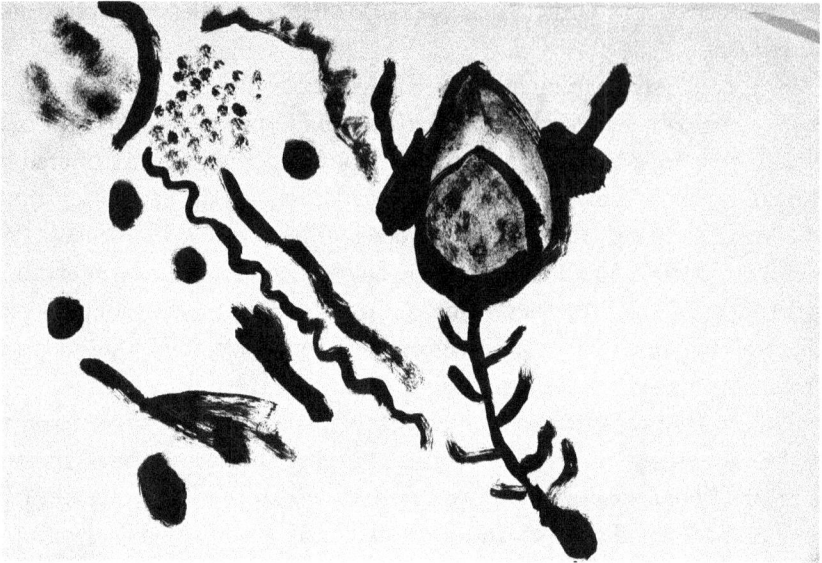

Figure 0.1 'A rose bud' replica artwork based on a painting by Peter 12 years.

Brief introduction to the authors of this book

Gita Ingram is an occupational therapist and graduate of the Therapeutic Skills with Children and Young people: Psychoanalytic Observation and Reflective Practice course at SIHR. This course was pivotal in providing her with a new lens through which she viewed her work. She is also a Systemic Practitioner. Following some years as Head Occupational Therapist in Lothian CAMHS, she led the looked after and accommodated children (LAAC) team, Edinburgh Connect, an innovative project jointly funded and managed by the Local Authority and the National Health Service (NHS). This experience, working with residential care units and with foster carers convinced her of the value of consultation, enhancing the skills and the understanding of those caring for traumatised children, either alongside individual therapy for children, or as a stand-alone therapeutic approach. A firm grasp of organisational dynamics underpins such work. Gita is currently working as an independent trainer and supervisor and has written about psychodynamic approaches and play in occupational therapy.

Susie Reade is an occupational therapist who was employed for 20 years in the trauma team in Lothian CAMHS. Her speciality was working with children who showed inappropriate sexual behaviour. Whilst intervention included family and systemic work, her passion was the direct individual work with children. She had undertaken training in psychoanalytic thinking at SIHR and she applied this to her use of individual child-led play as therapy. In addition, she devised imaginative educational methods of working with children on relational, sexual and body boundaries. Susie dovetailed into her employment a part-time degree in Art and Design, graduating in 2013. It is likely that the children with whom she worked in CAMHS were sensitive to her particular interest in their artwork. Hence, a few replicas of their paintings are printed in this publication. Susie herself continues to be an exhibiting artist. Continuing her interest in honest communication with children, however difficult that is, Susie is currently in her third year of learning British Sign Language, and she volunteers with a group of deaf children.

Annie Green is an occupational therapist, postgraduate in Counselling, who undertook the Infant Mental Health course at the SIHR which included a year-long baby observation. During her career in CAMHS Lothian she worked in a general outpatient team, the trauma team and for a number of years was head occupational therapist. Like her colleagues and fellow authors, her abiding interest has been the use of child-led play as an intervention with children who have experienced trauma. An important aspect of her management role in CAMHS was the training, support and supervision of occupational therapists within the model of play based occupational therapy, while steering and promoting the model through the waves of change and challenge within a busy CAMHS department. She now works as an exhibiting visual artist.

Reference list

Nicholls, L., Piergrossi, J.C., Gibertoni, C.de S & Daniel, M., eds. (2013). *Psychoanalytic Thinking in Occupational Therapy*. Wiley-Blackwell, pp. 105–127.

ACKNOWLEDGEMENTS

The anonymised children and their families with whom we have worked have taught us so much. Our biggest quota of thanks goes to them though they will not know that. Thank you also to our colleagues, friends and families who have been generous with their support and essential in the collaborative process to bring this book to fruition.

INTRODUCTION AND CHAPTER OUTLINES

In the sandpit Carrie played out a scene using the dinosaurs and a tiny plastic, tattered baby figure. The play was full of fear, violence and hopelessness. The room felt still around us, her focus intense, the play vivid and compelling. While I watched she made no sound, no eye contact and I sensed my very breath might interrupt. After what seemed like a long time, she scooped up the baby from its hiding place and wrapped her hand gently around it. She lifted her head to meet my eyes. At last, we had a connection, in which her silence eloquently conveyed a confusion of feelings and longing. It seemed too soon, too fragile for any words. Just as quickly the moment was gone and she swept an arm through the sand, scattering the dinosaurs and dismantling the scene as if it had never been there. We had begun….

The above excerpt beautifully illustrates an example of child-led therapy with Carrie. In observing Carrie closely during the session, the therapist recognised that Carrie was in her own world filled with fear and silence. Rather than actively encouraging an interaction, the therapist knew that she needed to stay with the child's silence allowing her to tiptoe (Music

DOI: 10.4324/9781003642862-1

2022) up to a connection with the therapist. When the child was ready, the therapist was there. They had made a therapeutic connection. This is the vital first step in working with children who present with complex trauma.

Child-led play and communication is a gentle approach which encourages relationship building for children who find relating hard. The vital foundations for this work are regularity, consistency, safety and confidentiality. Therapy can provide a way to think about events previously unthinkable and process the impact of such events through play and activity within the therapeutic relationship. This process may take just a few sessions to gain a good assessment of the child, or it may be the beginning of ongoing longer-term therapy.

The kitchen table provided the focal point for our discussions and for the writing of this book. We were a group of six occupational therapists who had worked together in Child and Adolescent Mental Health Services (CAMHS) for some years.

> We've just had a really interesting chat. Did anyone write it down?
> Can we continue to meet even if we don't actually write anything?
> Is this a leaflet? A paper? A chapter? A book?

These were some of the dilemmas we faced over the recent years of writing. In hindsight we recognised that the paper written by Susie Reade et al. (1999), 'Just Playing, is it time wasted?' formed a starting point. Now three of the original group have been able to take this project forward.

Referral to CAMHS is made for a myriad of difficulties including nightmares, flashbacks, dissociation, emotional regulation issues involving impulsivity, limited concentration, aggression and sexualised behaviour. Anxiety, overactivity, depression and self-harm may also be present. These difficulties may be symptoms of post-traumatic stress disorder (PTSD) or complex trauma (C-PTSD).

Underlying this presentation may be a cluster of developmental delays and deficits resulting from adverse early experiences. It is not surprising that these children are hard to reach emotionally. When a referral is received it is important to ask the question 'why now?' Frequently there have been concerns over a long period but something has tipped over an edge to make these concerns so urgent as to warrant a referral.

As occupational therapists in CAMHS, we provided assessment and treatment to children presenting with significant difficulties to support their emotional, sensory and environmental needs to help them manage their everyday lives. We worked closely with parents and professionals. Of significance to this book is the way we recognise the central role of play as the child's natural occupation. This approach has evolved to be known as play based occupational therapy (PBOT). Its purpose is to enhance the communication with traumatised children to help them process and understand what has happened to them.

In their survey of UK CAMHS occupational therapy practice, Brooks et al. (2018) found that most in their small sample of 27 therapists used therapeutic modalities of sensory processing and integration, cognitive behavioural therapies and systems and family therapies. Surprisingly all those in the survey used solely talking therapies with no play. This was in stark contrast to findings 35 years earlier (Jeffrey et al. 1984) that pointed to many therapists in CAMHS using play as their main therapeutic medium. This change may in part be due to the development and expansion in this period of Play Therapy as a profession. However, we believe that there continues to be a place within occupational therapy with children and young people, for play based assessment and intervention, thereby developing a skill set that makes us comfortable working in non-verbal ways with children who may not be able to use words to formulate or process their difficulties.

We define PBOT as a child-led approach using play for assessment and intervention which can enable children to communicate and indeed make links between internal/external worlds and past/present experiences. It is a way of helping children use their own language of play to communicate their problems and work through them (Blunden 2001). Engaging a child through play enables them to increase their own sense of agency. PBOT makes use of knowledge of child development, play activity, psychodynamic, humanist and attachment theories, communication and relational skills, sensory processing as well as generic multi-disciplinary skills in assessment, case and risk management and systemic working.

In this book, we aim to describe the application and theory of PBOT with children who present with complex trauma. By complex trauma we mean multiple experiences of ruptured close relationships which impact on a child's sense of safety and ability to develop on a healthy pathway.

Traumatic events might include direct experiences of abuse and neglect. Indirect traumatic experiences might include exposure to domestic violence and significant parental mental health and substance misuse issues. This may all take place against a background of disruptions of close attachment relationships. These lived experiences are often chronic so that such children may not have known anything different.

We have had a strong tradition within our occupational therapy team of practicing within a psychodynamic framework using child-led play and communication. This is often non-verbal. Whilst our practice has involved a variety of occupational therapy models, it is safe to say that it is the psychodynamic work that has most inspired and informed us over the years. Beyond occupational therapy, we were all fortunate to be able to undertake training in therapeutic skills with children through psychoanalytic observation and reflective practice courses. Colleagues from many disciplines have motivated us in sharing this way of working.

We recognise that in today's climate of increasing numbers of referrals of children to mental health services, current therapies often emphasise a quick fix approach. However, in our experience, for children with complex trauma, such therapeutic interventions are often not sufficient. Instead, more time intensive, most often weekly play based therapy is required where the therapeutic relationship is central to a child's recovery. These children cannot engage with brief interventions. The therapist drawing on good observational skills uses the self as a therapeutic tool to stay in the 'here and now' with the child, to take in their experience and think it through, so as to know how best to respond. This relationship and play based approach led by the child, forms an essential foundation for the shortest of therapeutic contact to the longest.

This book includes case studies and reflections of what happens in the therapeutic playroom. How do we observe and make sense of a child's communications? How do we as therapists recognise the feelings in the room and how do we respond? How are therapists affected by such work and what reflective support needs to be available to them? We wish to convey the highs and lows of therapy, the dilemmas, the hope, the fear, the confusion and the wonder that can all be part of the therapeutic relationship. It is hoped that this book might inspire clinicians and managers in CAMHS and other organisations to value direct observation and play based communication with troubled children. Whilst we are writing from an occupational therapy perspective, we anticipate that readers from other professional disciplines, such as psychology, social work, psychiatry, arts psychotherapy, play therapy, nursing and practitioners in the third sector will also find this book relevant to their practice with children and adolescents who have experienced complex trauma. It aims to be a practical and theoretical resource.

Most of our case studies are based on actual case material. We have made every effort to protect the children's anonymity by changing their names and distinguishing features. Some cases are a combination of several children known to us and some have almost taken on a life of their own. The meaning of what we have tried to convey has not been diluted. We have adapted children's drawings from clinical practice into replica illustrations for this book. Case examples are written from the therapist's perspective in the first person. Throughout this book the word 'parents' is used to mean the adults with the vital, close relationship with the child. The word 'carers' could equally well be used. The word 'children' includes young people.

Content and context of this book – chapter outlines

Chapter 1: Understanding complex trauma

We describe and define complex trauma as the profound disruptions in child development that can result from chronic experiences of abuse and neglect, a multitude of ruptured close relationships and moves of placement/home. To begin to understand such children, we need to ask not 'what is wrong with this child' but 'what has happened to this child'.

Research in the last 20 years has provided evidence of the impact these early experiences can have on brain development, and therefore on cognitive, social, emotional and physical development. Complex trauma is often pervasive over many generations. Whilst we acknowledge that trauma is cumulative and that different types of trauma overlap, a major part of this chapter addresses how different types of traumas affect a child's developing sense of self and identity. This is illustrated by brief case material.

Chapter 2: Additional vulnerabilities to trauma

In this chapter, we consider four out of several possible groups of children who are particularly vulnerable to the effects of trauma. These include child refugees, children who are exposed to harmful internet online content, children who identify with gender dysphoria and children who may present as neurodivergent. Their experiences often overlap with situations leading to trauma. We explain how presentations of complex trauma can be frequently compounded by co-existing situations and conditions which are not caused by trauma, but which can have significant effects on a child's development and require support in their own right. In addition, these children may have grown up in unsettled and traumatising environments which exacerbate their existing difficulties. We describe how important it is to focus on the detail of any therapeutic response with the child and the family in order that it is carefully tailored to their situation and need.

Chapter 3: Play as communication and as a child's natural occupation

Play is a child's natural occupation and is of central importance to the physical, emotional and social development of the growing individual. It forms the basis of much therapeutic work with children. In this chapter, we explore play as a means of expression through different developmental stages, from babyhood through to adolescence and beyond. We consider what play actually is, why it is so important and the reasons why some children are unable to play. We look at adults' attitudes to children's play and how parents and professionals may need support to be comfortable with child-led play. The chapter leads into considering the use of play as therapy including occupational therapy, which we fully explore in later sections of this book. Writers through the ages have explored the meaning of play and some of their thoughts will be quoted throughout this section to support the material.

Chapter 4: What happens in the playroom

In this chapter, we look at practical ways of engaging with individual children through child-led therapy. We discuss ways to set up a therapeutic playroom and to create a safe space for emotional exploration. The reader's understanding of this process is enhanced through brief case studies which highlight ways that children communicate through play and how the therapeutic relationship is formed and used. Opportunities for therapeutic intervention and how to manage challenging situations are considered. This includes the therapist being tuned into their own emotional responses in the therapeutic encounter. The therapist's management of time, space and self all contribute to a sense of containment for the entire therapeutic experience. Finally, we give some examples of how the therapeutic contact can be extended to the use of letters, phone calls and video calls with children.

Chapter 5: Assessment, review and planning

We outline the assessment process using PBOT. A combination of child-led play and some activities structured by the therapist may be used. Gathering information about the child from a variety of sources – family, school, social work and any other relevant agencies, is important at this stage. Following this process, the review and planning of the next steps may lead to several outcomes, including ongoing therapy with the child, indirect contact with the parents and professionals only, referral for another therapeutic modality or discharge. We discuss how to share information from a child's sessions with parents and professionals, including dilemmas over respecting the child's privacy. We present a detailed case study to demonstrate the process.

Chapter 6: Theoretical underpinning of play based occupational therapy

Therapists need a theoretical framework to guide their work. The theoretical base for PBOT is wide ranging. Here we highlight the importance of developing an observational stance and a reflective pattern of practice, regardless of theoretical position. We consider the impact of the child's earliest experiences on their development. We explore the influences of psychoanalytic, neurodevelopmental, person-centred, and systemic theories. This leads into thinking about the practical applications of a firm theoretical base, including therapists being tuned into not just their clients' responses, but equally importantly to their own countertransference reactions. We describe the Vivaio (MOVI) Occupational Therapy model (Piergrossi and Gibertini 2013), which is informed by psychoanalysis and the parallels between PBOT and MOVI.

Chapter 7: The therapeutic process

In this chapter, we consider how the therapeutic relationship progresses over time and how opportunities for emotional growth at different stages of therapy can emerge. The beginning phase is about establishing trust that can, over time, withstand challenging periods in therapy. The vital foundations for this work are regularity, consistency, safety and confidentiality. The middle part is when the real work takes place. Here we may find progress hard to gauge. Sessions may be challenging, and we may struggle to know how to proceed. This is when themes begin to emerge, and transformative things can happen. Ending therapy must be thought about from the start. Ending therapy in a planned and thoughtful way can give the child an opportunity to experience a transition where feelings of rejection and abandonment can be worked through.

The main part of this chapter consists of two case studies to highlight beginnings, middles and endings of therapy. We consider situations which have been particularly difficult for the therapist to manage. Although both children have experienced complex trauma, the themes of their play are remarkably different.

Chapter 8: Working with the multidisciplinary team

We discuss the role of occupational therapists in the multidisciplinary team in CAMHS. This includes a review of work with the individual child, their family and the professional network. How do occupational therapists collaborate with other members of the clinical team and with the network that forms the team around the child? How does joint work and cross-fertilisation of ideas and knowledge contribute to the whole experience for the child and their family? We address issues to do with disclosures and working within child protection guidelines. We cover systemic and wider socio-political issues that impact on working with children with complex trauma and their families in CAMHS. We conclude with an extended description of multidisciplinary consultation to the adults involved with a child in the care system, aiming to enhance the consultees' understanding of the inner world of the child.

Chapter 9: Supervision and support

In this chapter, we argue that clinical supervision is essential for those practising therapy with children. The supervisory relationship aims to support the personal and professional growth of therapists and to ensure that therapy can progress safely. A case study is used to demonstrate this process. There is a role for supervision to explore both internal and external factors that support the therapy. The therapist needs to hold an 'internal space' to contain and process the child's communications. External factors located in the family and in the wider system contribute to a robust base from which the child has permission to engage in therapeutic exploration. Here we think about the need for a supportive culture within the organisation. We describe a CAMHS department-wide reflective practice group, which enhanced therapeutic skills and professional confidence.

Reference list

Blunden, P. (2001). The therapeutic use of play. In Lougher, L. ed. *Occupational Therapy for Child and Adolescent Mental Health*. Churchill Livingstone, pp. 67–86.

Brooks, R., Monro, S., Jones, J. (2018). Occupational therapy in children and young people's mental health: A UK survey of Practice. *Royal College of Occupational Therapists Specialist Section for Children, Young People and Families Journal*, 22(1), 9–15

Jeffrey, L.I.H., Lyne, S.C., Redfern, F. (1984). Child and adolescent psychiatry – Survey 1984. *British Journal of Occupational Therapy*, 47 (12), 370–372.

Music, G. (2022). *Respark: Igniting Spark and Joy after Trauma and Depression*. Mind-Nurturing Books, p. 30.

Reade, S., Hunter, H., McMillan, I.R. (1999). Just playing … is it time wasted? *British Journal of Occupational Therapy*, 62 (4), 157–162.

1

UNDERSTANDING COMPLEX TRAUMA

This book concerns children with many serious difficulties. They are often angry and impulsive, frightened and frightening, controlling and demanding. They are watchful, suspicious and unable to trust. They may be withdrawn and cut themselves off from others or their behaviours may be overfamiliar and sexualised. They may soil and wet, they may overeat or not eat. They may self-harm and threaten suicide. They can seem like a threatened frightened animal that needs to growl and attack and keep everyone at bay.

To begin to understand such children, we need to ask not 'what is wrong with this child' but 'what has happened to this child'.

The word trauma originates from the Greek word 'trauma' meaning 'wound' or to 'pierce'.

Maté and Maté (2024) have famously said that trauma is what happens inside you as a result of what has happened to you. We would expand that to include what has not happened to you, what have you been deprived of and what basic needs have you missed out on.

DOI: 10.4324/9781003642862-2

Joanne Stubley, in her book *Complex Trauma* (2022, p. 11) draws together definitions of trauma, all of which stress the inescapable, overwhelming helplessness, terror and dread caused by long-term abuse. Such experiences affect the entire being, the physical, the psychological, the relational and the social aspects of a child's life.

The term Complex Trauma was used by Herman (1992) to describe a constellation of symptoms that occurred following chronic, repetitive and prolonged trauma. However, it was not until 2019 that the term Complex Trauma was included in ICD-11 (The 11th edition of the International Classificatory System of Diseases [ICD-11] 2019) as Complex Post-Traumatic Stress Disorder (C-PTSD). This disorder is interchangeable with the terms Complex Trauma or Developmental Trauma.

'Developmental trauma disorder', as proposed by Van der Kolk (2005) extends the concept of complex trauma into a meaningful categorisation of the wide range of developmental difficulties and deficits that can be seen in children and young people. These include affective, physiological, attentional and behavioural dysregulation, PTSD symptoms and functional impairment in learning, cognition, communication, relationships and general health.

Multiple experiences of trauma and frequently ruptured close relationships impact on a child's sense of safety and ability to develop on a healthy pathway. Traumatic events might include repeated experiences of abuse including neglect, sexual abuse, significant attachment disruptions, exposure to domestic violence and significant parental mental health or substance misuse issues. These experiences can often occur within wide family groups and across generations and have become part of the culture within which the child grows up. They need to be considered in the context of societal issues such as poverty and poor housing. The frequently chronic nature of such experiences means that the children may not have known anything different in their lives. Often the children are in the care system, where further experiences of placement loss and disruption compound the issues.

The mitigating effect of consistent attachment relationships has often been disrupted or unavailable for these children. This in turn makes new attachments difficult to form. Figure 1.1 suggests a natural fit between child and adult as well as a space.

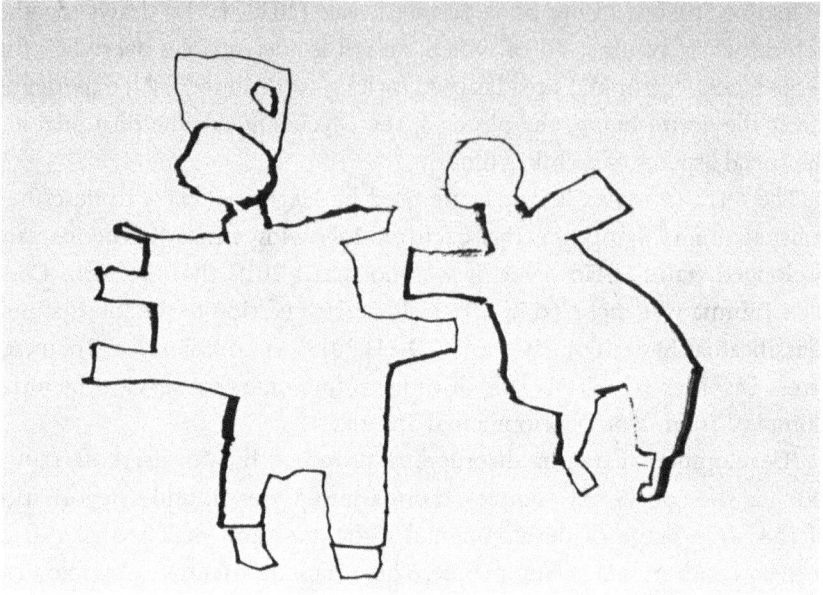

Figure 1.1 'Me and my foster mum' replica artwork based on a drawing by Stephanie 9 years.

Literature around Adverse Childhood Experiences (ACES) (Felitti and Anda 2010) has been helpful in giving all of us across children's services a way of thinking and communicating about the impact of such experiences on development throughout the lifespan.

Impact of complex trauma on formation of a sense of self and on identity

Children suffering from complex trauma often develop coping strategies such as fight, flight or freeze behaviours such as dissociation and numbing, in order to defend themselves against overwhelming anxiety and literally in order to survive. Such strategies may come at a heavy cost to the development of a sense of self. We'll consider some of the specific features of different forms of abuse, whilst acknowledging that much abuse is cumulative and cannot be considered in isolation. A child who has been sexually abused is also likely to have been neglected and emotionally abused. Children who have been abused in one way are more vulnerable to other forms of abuse.

Neglect

Whereas abuse indicates that something bad has happened or is happening to a child, neglect refers to an absence of nurturing input. The psychoanalyst and paediatrician Donald Winnicott, who coined the term 'good enough parent', suggested that, in good enough infant–parent relationships, when a baby looks at his mother's face, the baby sees himself (1971, p. 112). This is the basis, over time, of the young child developing a sense of who they are. Identity is formed during the early years from millions of everyday interactions where, for most of the time, the child can be seen and thought about for who they are. It follows that when such caregiving is missing the consequences can be devastating.

As Graham Music (2011, p. 205) writes:

> Neglected children have not had an experience of a parent sensitive to their bodily and emotional states, who psychologically holds and imitates them, and is attuned to their gestures.... nor do they have anyone to help them with anxious or frightening moments. Their signals are not read by others....Neglected children often do not believe that they can have an impact on others....they often live in a flat and desultory world.

Such children become vulnerable to further abuse. Neglectful families struggle to protect their children from dangers. The children can become desperately needy for closeness at any cost. Yet they may not recognise a trusting relationship or expect protection. Music (2009) has described children who have suffered chronic neglect and trauma as 'undrawn', as opposed to 'withdrawn' (indicating something to withdraw from). In his book *Respark* (2022), Music points to such reactions being whole body responses affecting metabolism and muscle tone, leading to damped down, slowed down states or states of tension and hyper-arousal.

Sexual abuse

Sexual abuse is an assault on the entire being, on the self, both physically and emotionally. Children are asked not to trust their own feelings and may be told that experiences which are frightening and painful are in fact a game that they may be privileged to play. Their feelings don't count and don't tally with their experiences. As Margaret Hunter (2001, p. 91) describes there is an assault on the victim's truth, on the victim's reality. She points to the most troubling aspect of sexual abuse being the deception and manipulation that these children are subjected to, alongside the physical assault. She advocates conceptualising sexual abuse primarily in relationship terms. Children who have been sexually abused often talk about having to 'step outside of their body', to dissociate in order to survive. They are often forced to cover up the abuse by lying (at times under threat) and can end up building complicated webs around such lying, to the point when they themselves feel complicit in the abuse, feeling 'this is our secret, and I can belong and identify with it'. Such loyalty is hidden to the outside world and is often accompanied with feelings of shame. Even though they want the abuse to stop, it may perversely meet a neglected child's need for intimacy. This maybe the only closeness they know so they are held in a terrible bind. Their early intrusive experience of sexual contact can leave them with little idea of what safe, predictable physical and emotional closeness can be like. Children may have little understanding of ordinary relationships and boundaries with either adults or other children and their behaviours may become sexualised. Their sense of self becomes confused and skewed. It is not difficult to appreciate therefore the far-reaching effects on children's ability to manage everyday life and to trust and build new relationships.

For Simon, the sexual abuse many years ago felt immediate and as a physical presence in his body:

Simon aged 10 was referred following multiple rape by a family friend. He was now living with foster carer Liz and had no contact with his family. In sessions up till now he had fluctuated between risk taking behaviour on the stairs on the way to the therapy room and lying down on the floor hiding his face. For this seventh session he asked Liz to join him for a while. In her presence he drew a large blue shape and scribbled to fill its centre. I said how I wonder if he's been planning what he wants to think about today. He then said rapidly how really angry he feels because 'I was raped, and he got away with it. He wasn't locked up. He locked me in a room and tied me up.' Liz held him and hugged him. The room was quiet. Liz explained she would leave the room now and would be in the waiting room. I asked him 'When you think about those rapes, where in your body do you feel that?'

He replied, 'in my belly' and he rubbed his belly.

I asked, 'How big is that feeling out of a score one to ten?'

He replied, 'ten.' He stood up and drummed his hands on the table. I asked him if he wanted me to join the drumming. He did. I drummed my hands next to his. We drummed at different speeds, mirroring each other. I said this drumming might help sort some of this out. He continued with the drumming getting louder and using the weight of his whole body. He suddenly stopped and said, 'It all happened a long time ago and now it isn't happening'. He moved on to play in the sand.

Physical abuse and domestic violence

Unlike sexual abuse, physical child abuse has been known about throughout history, although the extent of it has not been recognised until the last century. Lanyado (2018, pp. 19–20) points to the deliberate harming of children by their parents and others coming to light in 1950s as 'the battered child syndrome'. Understanding has since grown about the many sadistic ways that children can be injured, particularly if those who harm them are the same people who are meant to protect them. Abuse can sometimes come to light spontaneously in play sessions with children, as with Stephanie (Figure 1.2).

Recent years have seen several Child Abuse Public Inquiries into deaths of children such as Baby P in 2007 and Victoria Climbie in 2000. In spite of recommendations which include a fundamental reappraisal of child protection services and how they work together, child cruelty continues often unnoticed and below the radar and children continue to die at the hands of their parents. This was the case recently of ten-year-old Sara Sharif who died in August 2023. During the court case against members of her family, Sara was reported in the press (The Guardian 2024) as coming across as happy and bubbly 'still doing her best to be a child', whilst beaten black and blue under her clothes and with visible injuries such as a piece of her finger missing.

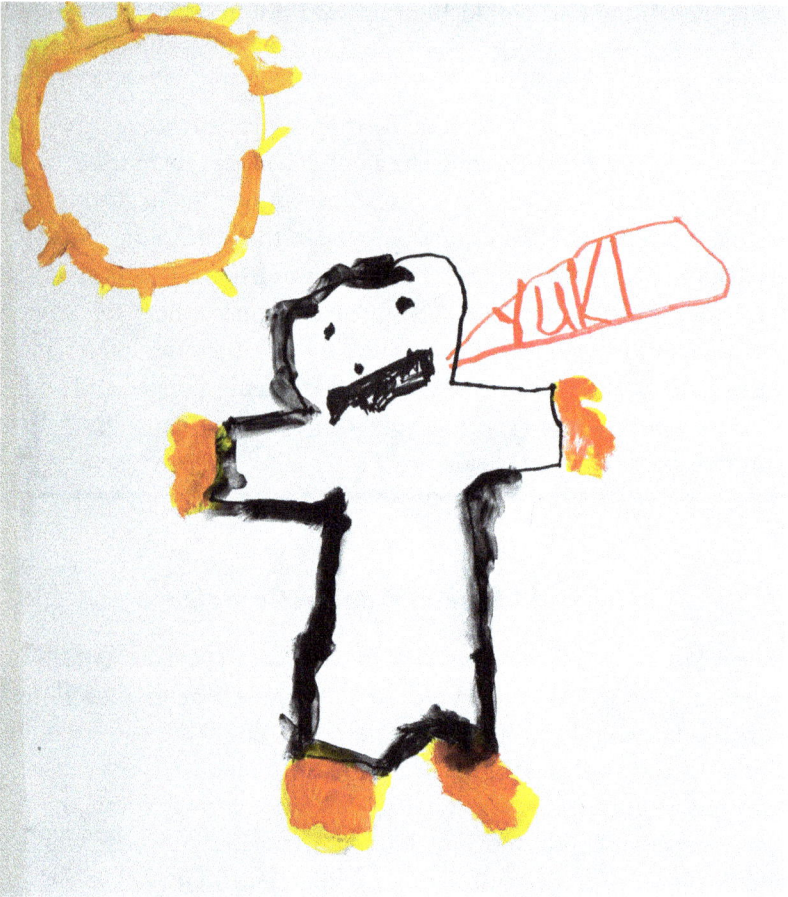

Figure 1.2 'Me being made to eat something horrible' replica artwork based on a painting by Stephanie 9 years.

Growing up in a violent environment may mean that children have to put aside their own needs and emotions and 'lie low' in order not to aggravate further abuse or even to survive. Fear and anger may have to be hidden. There is little space for spontaneity. Such children are often hyper-vigilant and with a strong urge to conform and please. Their unmet needs may emerge in fears and anxieties, sleep difficulties, nightmares, wetting, soiling and smearing.

Domestic violence causes trauma, whether or not the physically violent acts happen amongst adults or are directed at the child. Indeed, to witness or hear a parent being repeatedly threatened or harmed by another adult has serious effects on children.

In addition to children having to remain hyper-alert for their own protection, feelings of powerlessness and guilt at not being able to stop the abuse and protect a parent are common. Shame and a feeling that they need to keep what they know quiet even though they want the abuse to stop, is a significant dilemma for children. They may attempt to silence younger siblings. Again, such children are often drawn into webs of family secrets and lies with all the associated issues to do with trust and loyalty. In their efforts to protect the abused parent the child may struggle to have an identity of their own. Alternatively, they may reject all their own vulnerability and unconsciously identify with the aggressor through violent behaviour or sexually harmful behaviour, with devastating consequences.

Is this the case for Leah, was she hurting her own vulnerable self?

Leah aged 9 was in foster care, her brother having returned to the care of their parents. Leah took the baby doll out of the cot. She attempted to change the baby's nappy by wrapping a paper towel around her. She couldn't make it stay in place and repeatedly tried to fix it, becoming increasing frustrated but not asking for help from me. She shouted at the baby, blaming the baby for the difficulty. The scene ended with Leah punching the baby in the face and asking to finish the session.

Parental addiction and serious mental health difficulties

Whilst these are separate issues that may or may not overlap, it seems appropriate to consider their effects on children's growing identity together. It is worth stressing that there are many parents who suffer from mental health issues who are also fully able to be protective and caring parents. Here we are referring to those whose mental health issues are so serious that they significantly impact on their ability to parent safely. Equally we are referring to those suffering from debilitating addictions.

The overwhelming struggle for many children living with adults who are addicted to drugs or alcohol is the unpredictability, volatility and the adult's preoccupation above all with 'getting the next hit'. Children's needs become a low priority. Parents may be violent and frightening one moment and loving and caring another. They are often unavailable emotionally to their children.

Those parents suffering from severe depression may shut down and rely on the children to take care of the household and younger siblings. One mother incorporated her child in her psychotic delusional state and projected her fears of attack onto the child, who she thought was about to harm her. Both with addictions and serious mental health problems children tend to become parental, taking on responsibilities far beyond their age. This can influence their school attendance and their ability to develop interests and relationships outside of the family. They may be involved in procuring the drugs or 'stealing' alcohol or food. They often feel that they must hide what is happening at home lest they be removed from their parents' care. They may feel in the middle, between their parents and outside agencies trying to help. They become hyper-alert to their parents' moods. Such children can become fearful, hypervigilant, overly independent and controlling. Allowing their own feelings to be seen or known can be dangerous.

Emotional abuse

Emotional abuse is an inherent part of all form of abuse. It is present in the repetitions and rupturing of relationships in complex trauma. According to Boulton and Hindle (2000, p. 441), it is hard to imagine neglect, physical or sexual abuse without there being an emotional component to it. They argue that the emotional aspects of the abuse can have the most damaging long-term effect on a child's development and sense of self. The National Guidance for Child Protection in Scotland (2023) includes the following:

> Emotional abuse is persistent emotional neglect or ill treatment that has severe and persistent adverse effects on a child's emotional development. It may involve conveying to a child that they are worthless or unloved, inadequate or valued only in so far as they meet the needs of another person. It may involve the imposition of age or developmentally inappropriate expectations on a child. It may involve repeated silencing, ridiculing or intimidation. It may involve causing children to feel frightened or in danger or exploiting or corrupting children. It may involve seeing or hearing the abuse of another. Some level of emotional abuse is present in all types of ill treatment of a child; it can also occur independently of other forms of abuse.

Glaser (2002) provides a helpful conceptual framework for understanding and assessing emotional abuse. It underlines the persistent negative attitudes towards the child, the emotional unavailability to the child and the failure to recognise the child's individuality and psychological boundaries.

Harmful or inappropriate sexual behaviour in children

A devastating and potentially far-reaching consequence of growing up in violent, sexualised and abusive environments is that children may develop inappropriate or harmful sexual behaviours. The juxtaposition of the word child with the word sex is a disparity. It reflects the breaking down of boundaries, an abuse of power and a skewed sense of what it means to be a child. According to McNeish and Scott (2023), the term 'harmful sexual behaviours' describes:

> a continuum of behaviours displayed by children and young people under 18, ranging from those considered 'inappropriate' at a particular age or developmental stage to 'problematic ', 'abusive' and 'violent' behaviours.
>
> (p. 2)

Inappropriate sexual behaviour is likely to occur in young children who may have been sexually abused or exposed to inappropriate sexual material face to face or online, or who have grown up in highly sexualised environments. In older children who display harmful or violent sexual behaviour, research has shown a link with experiences of neglect, physical or sexual abuse, witnessing domestic violence or having parents with mental health or substance abuse issues (McNeish and Scott 2023). As mentioned in the previous section, children often have little choice but to identify with the aggressor. Even when a child is removed from the sexualised environment, they may continue to idealise their family and deny their own vulnerability. Thus, harmful sexual behaviour may continue in their care placement.

It is however important to note that

> most victims of sexual abuse do not go on to abuse others and that most children and young people who display sexually harmful behaviours do not go on to sexually offend as adults. However, older adolescents who abuse younger children, and those whose sexual behaviours involve violence, are at greater risk of further sexual offending.
>
> (p. 4)

Several case studies in the following chapters describe therapy with children who have been referred because of sexual abuse about which the child continues to be significantly disturbed and confused. Therapy with children who present with sexually harmful behaviours is also described.

Concluding thoughts

When considering different types of abuse individually and collectively, it is not hard to understand how most children meeting the criteria for complex trauma also show characteristics of Disorganised Insecure Attachment, as described by Ainsworth (1978). Often the child is placed in a precarious dilemma when the person who is there to protect them is also the person who abuses them, either directly or by failing to keep them from harm. Often, we do not know exactly what has happened to a child.

What can we learn from Alice about her likely experiences and attachment patterns, and can the following observation inform how we might try to engage with her?

Alice aged 8, in foster care, was referred following likely abuse and neglect. Her speech was hard to understand but her play was full of urgency and action as if she needed to make up for lost time. Little emotion was apparent. She seemed to over or under express emotion. When an opportunity to voice disappointment emerged, such as when her sandcastle collapsed, she did not express this. At that moment she said, 'the sand is dead'. Often the toy animals were described as being on the run and 'everyone is getting hurt'. Human figures were shown to be confusing e.g. rescuers killed those they had just saved. Fights resulted in burials. Alice became so involved with her play that she could be breathless and gasping for air. She seemed to expect adults to die or kill and showed hyper-vigilance as a result, keeping watch to ensure her own survival.

Careful observation of how a child presents, in addition to reading case histories and chronologies, can help us extrapolate what may have happened to them. It is then important to consider the impacts of different forms of abuse when we consider how best to understand these children and try to reach them therapeutically.

Reference list

Ainsworth, M.D.S. (1978). *Patterns of Attachment: A Psychological Study of the Strange Situation.* Lawrence Erlbaum Associates, Inc.

Boulton, S., Hindle, D. (2000). Emotional abuse: The work of a multidisciplinary consultation group in a child psychiatric service. *Clinical Child Psychology and Psychiatry,* 5 (3), 439–452.

Felitti, V.J., Anda, R.F. (2010). The relationship of adverse childhood experiences to adult medical disease, psychiatric disorders and sexual behaviour: Implications for healthcare. In Lanius, R.A., Vermetten, E., Pain, C. eds. *The Impact of Early Life Trauma on Health and Disease: The Hidden Epidemic.* Cambridge University Press, pp. 245–258.

Glaser, D. (2002). Emotional abuse and neglect: A conceptual framework. *Child Abuse and Neglect,* 26, 697–714.

Herman, J.L. (1992). Complex PTSD: A syndrome in survivors of prolonged and repeated trauma. *Journal of Traumatic Stress,* 5 (3), 377–391.

Hunter, M. (2001). *Psychotherapy with Young People in Care: Lost and Found.* Brunner-Routledge.

ICD-11. (2019). *International Classification of Diseases.* 11the Revision. World Health Organisation.

Lanyado, M. (2018). *Transforming Despair to Hope: Reflections on the Psychotherapeutic Process with Severely Neglected and Traumatised Children.* Routledge.

Maté, G., Maté, D. (2024). *The Myth of Normal: Illness, Health and Healing in a Toxic Culture.* Vermilion.

McNeish, D., Scott, S. (2023). Key messages from research on children and young people who display harmful sexual behaviour. In *Centre of Expertise on Child Sexual Abuse* (2nd, pp. 1–16). https://doi.org/10.47117/NNXP7141, www.csacentre.org.uk.

Music, G. (2009). Neglecting neglect: Some thoughts about children who have lacked good input, and are 'undrawn' and 'unenjoyed'. *Journal of Child Psychotherapy,* 35 (2), 142–156.

Music, G. (2011). *Nurturing Natures: Attachment and Children's Emotional, Sociocultural and Brain Development.* Psychology Press, p. 205.

Music, G. (2022). *Respark: Igniting Spark and Joy after Trauma and Depression.* Mind-Nurturing Books.

Scottish Government. (2023). *National guidance for Child Protection in Scotland 2021 – Updated 2023.* Scottish Government Publications.

Stubley, J. (2022). Complex trauma: The initial consultation. In Stubley, J., Young, L. eds. *Complex Trauma: The Tavistock Model.* Routledge, pp. 11–33.

The Guardian. (11.12.2024). *Sara Sharif Was Doing Her Best to Be a Child.* Guardian News and Media, Guardian Media Group.

Van der Kolk, B.A. (2005). Developmental trauma disorder: Toward a rational diagnosis for children with complex trauma histories. *Psychiatric Annals,* 35 (5), 401–408.

Winnicott, D.W. (1971). *Playing and Reality.* Routledge.

2

ADDITIONAL VULNERABILITIES TO TRAUMA

This chapter covers circumstances where children are particularly vulnerable to the effects of trauma. A significant number of these children are referred to Child and Adolescent Mental Health Services (CAMHS). We have chosen just four out of several possible groups of children: child refugees, children exposed to harmful online content, children who identify as transgender and children who are neurodivergent. Their experiences often overlap with situations leading to complex trauma. They may have grown up in traumatising environments which exacerbate their existing difficulties or they may experience their current circumstances as traumatic per se.

Trauma and child refugees

There have been an increasing number of referrals in recent years of child refugees, some of whom live with their families and may be seeking asylum, some who have lost their families and are now in care. They may have been trafficked. These children all have experienced perilous journeys and

DOI: 10.4324/9781003642862-3

many have witnessed unspeakable traumas, including losing members of their own family in terrible circumstances. They will be suffering from post-traumatic stress disorder. They may be marginalised in their new country and experience prejudice. The task of assimilating into a new society, often with a new language is in itself a challenge. Nevertheless, they are a heterogeneous group. Whereas in some cases traumatisation will be lifelong, many have grown up in supportive families and have developed secure attachments and inner resources prior to the violence and upheaval that led to them fleeing their country. This is quite unlike most of the children suffering from complex trauma in this country. When a referral for a child refugee is received it is therefore important to try and acquire as much detailed information as possible (acknowledging that we often may not know all the facts) about the external world of the child now and prior to coming to this country, including the political and practical situation (Melzak 1999). The detail of our responses will be carefully tailored. Some children require direct trauma therapy. In many cases, significant adults may need some help initially in assessing and disentangling the child's experience from their own response to these experiences and time to assess what the child's needs may be (Melzak 1999, p. 427). Rahim is an example of this.

How might we think about the following observation of Rahim?

Rahim aged 11 had arrived as a refugee from a middle eastern country. He had been without close family members during several months in another country and it was not clear with whom he had travelled. Currently he lived with foster carers whilst his family was being tracked down. At school he was very quiet though his English language was adequate. He spent much time alone. He ate very little and was underweight. He had told his teacher that he made a mistake at a border crossing by going to sleep and then losing his family. It was his fault. He feared his parents wouldn't want him anymore.

Rahim was accompanied to his first assessment session by his carers. He was small and thin. He didn't want to take off his jacket. He pulled his hood down over his face so that he couldn't see or be seen. It felt to me as though he wanted to be invisible.

He examined a reel of sticky tape, finding the end and trying to stick his own fingers to the table. His carer accidentally dropped some coins on the floor. He immediately undid the sticky tape, picked up the coins and lay down on the floor under a blanket. His carers encouraged him to draw but he stayed hidden. To sit too near him on the floor felt intrusive to me. Connection was difficult and I felt his hopelessness and vulnerability. The session seemed too painful for him, and we agreed to cut it short and that the adults would continue to meet in the first instance. I realised when he left, that he hadn't spoken one word.

Trauma and the internet

Social media and gaming online provide many hours of interest for children currently. When used responsibly, the internet can be a wonderful source of knowledge and provide endless opportunities for education and creativity. When clinicians try to understand children's presentations, it is crucial that they explore their access to and use of the internet.

Nevertheless, the downsides for children's use of the internet are becoming increasingly evident in today's society. It is common for primary aged children to have access to social media and mobile devices, when the internet can be used away from home without adequate supervision. Much of the material that they access is potentially harmful. A study in 2023 for the Children's Commissioner for England found that a quarter of 16–21-year-olds first saw pornography on the internet while still at primary school. By the age of 13, 50% had been exposed to it (BBC News 31.01.2023). Some of the content is violent. Social media can be highly addictive and can lead some children to live almost exclusively in this artificial, lonely world with little connection to real life around them. This can take them to some very dark places where they are vulnerable to unsafe content, including signposting to self-harming, committing suicide and harming others.

Parents may do their best to monitor their child's internet use, but their children can be more skilled than them. Attempts by Governments to legislate for online safety and age restrictions are important developments but risk lagging behind technological advances.

Internet forums are also ideal for paedophiles to access children. They might befriend, groom, demand indecent photos and use blackmail to ensure their practice can continue. Online child abuse has expanded significantly in the last 25 years and spread worldwide. Photos are often the currency used in online child abuse.

Samantha aged 10 was referred due to a deterioration of her behaviour. Her early history was of disrupted relationships, 3 foster placements before her adoption aged 5. Her adoptive parents described her presentation until she was 9 years old as anxious, shy and having difficulty identifying her emotions. However, she enjoyed sports, football and swimming in particular, painting and cooking. Parents found that if they joined her in her chosen activity, she was less anxious and could talk a little about her feelings. For the past year her parents noted a worrying change in her behaviour, when she spent increasing amounts of time alone in her bedroom, refusing to go to any sports, avoiding any cooking and easily becoming tearful.

Her parents said they checked her internet use once a week. Despite this her older brother alerted parents to online chat she was having with 'another 10-year-old'. He had noticed that this 'peer's' photo showed a young man. Parents alerted services and investigation by child protection services found that for the past year she had been sending photos to the man, some of which were indecent. He had demanded this of her and threatened that if she told anyone he would find where she lived and take her away. There was a police investigation which revealed the young man's vast collection of indecent images of children. At the time of writing, it was not clear if he might have sold images of Samantha along with images of other children. The police will continue to stay in contact with the family as the effect of this on Samantha could be devastating.

The referral to CAMHS had occurred before the online abuse came to light. However, this became the focus of our intervention as it was likely that the abuse might explain some of Samantha's changed behaviour. It was decided that we would offer support to Samantha's parents. As a result, they tightened their monitoring of internet use. They increased the time they spent with her on other activities. They helped her to speak about her feelings which included the man making her feel really special, and she now missed that. Also, he had made her feel extremely frightened, with the blackmailing, threats and secrecy. Gradually Samantha returned to her sports activities and became interested in making clay animals.

Samantha's story is quite contained, the online abuse was discovered and acted upon. There may still be further effects on Samantha, as she matures. She may need individual support at that stage. However, this demonstrates the ease by which children can be exploited and the importance of being alert to children's changing behaviours.

Trauma and gender dysphoria

In our CAMHS practice, we accepted referrals for children who expressed, in various ways, a wish to be different. Thinking and vocabulary about gender issues have proliferated in society as a whole and clinically. There has been a significant increase in referrals of adolescent onset gender dysphoria. The speed of this shift has made it challenging for everyone to adapt and understand what this really means for children and young people and how clinicians can offer interventions that are helpful. Gender Dysphoria is a relatively recently named condition, having replaced Gender Identity Disorder in DSM-5 (The fifth edition of the Diagnostic and Statistical Manual of Mental Disorders [DSM-5] 2013). This shift reflects a change from considering a *disorder* to exploring an *identity*, meaning that we are engaging in a developmental process (Lemma 2022).

According to Ann Horne (2023), gender may be an explanatory framework which shrouds other difficulties, such as severe neglect, anxiety and depression, deliberate self-harm and social isolation or being a victim of bullying. Autism, especially in girls, is overrepresented. In our experience many children referred to our sexual trauma team expressed a wish to change gender as a direct result of the abuse they suffered. In simple terms, 13-year-old Mandy, now known as Michael, felt vulnerable to further abuse as a girl and felt safer when identifying as a boy. Many writers (Horne 2023; Lemma 2023) have noted that a wish to transition often is less about moving towards a different gender than moving away from something that feels deeply wrong and uncomfortable at the level of the embodied self. Understandably, these children want to look forward, not back. Coming back to Michael, they constructed their new identity in terms of dress, use of pronouns and social identity. Their environment at home and at school was adapting to this, and any reference to their pre-transitioning life was avoided.

In our opinion this is not without problems. Lemma (2023) approaches this in a balanced way

> Our natal body is for all of us an unavoidable part of our narrative and identity no matter how we might later choose to modify it.
>
> (p. 81)

Some children wish to refer to their pre-transition name as their 'dead name', representing a dead part of themselves. However, an important part of transitioning is being able to reflect on what it means to be transgender. Lemma (2023) has written about using pre-transitioning photographs with young people to gradually help them integrate the different parts of themselves into their life narrative. For some young people therapy is more about dealing with the trauma they have experienced, and the concern about gender identity might become a side issue.

This is a very heterogeneous group of children, and even though this one issue may be at the forefront for the young person and their family, it tells us very little about what is going on for them and what they are struggling with. In today's climate where gender issues have become so politicised, it is difficult to approach this work in an open way. However, as with any young person, we need to meet them as an individual and learn about their particular issues with compassion and curiosity.

This was also the case with Ali, for whom the level of distress and inner turmoil was clear:

Ali aged 15 had had several referral episodes since the age of 9, due to low mood, accounts of bullying and self-harm. The current referral was due to anxiety, increasing self-harm by burning and suicidal thoughts and plans. They felt stuck and sick of themselves having to live as person they didn't like. Ali considered themselves non-binary.

In the initial assessment session Ali spoke of not wanting to be in this body, wanting to be taller, have a deeper voice and how they look better in male clothing. They told me they were exclusively attracted to females. Puberty was the worst thing that ever happened, and they wanted to rip off their breasts. They felt stuck in their body and wouldn't be happy until their body died. They felt a burden to their family, but they didn't want to get better as the body 'skin suit' would still be there. Ali was wondering what was wrong with them, whether they have bi-polar, depression, autism and whether they are trans? They try to explain how they feel but other people don't understand.

This book is of course about the use of play as therapy. Ali is beyond the age where play might be the obvious choice of intervention. However, they may be interested in using paint and other creative media as a way of expressing themself. Although the referral did not mention any abuse or trauma, clinicians would need to keep an open mind.

Trauma and neurodivergence

Presentations of complex trauma can be frequently compounded by co-existing conditions which are not caused by trauma, but which can have significant effects on a child's development and require support in their own right. These include neurodevelopmental conditions such as autism, attention deficit hyperactivity disorder (ADHD), Tourette's syndrome, dyspraxia and sensory processing disorder. These all come under the umbrella term of neurodivergence. Some of the presenting difficulties of such neurodivergence are similar to the behaviours we see in neurotypical children who have suffered complex trauma. Symptoms of extreme anxiety, self-harm, difficulty with sleeping and eating, dysregulation and dissociation are common for both groups. Peer relationships tend to be challenging for all these children who in different ways struggle with communicating.

Since one does not rule out the other it can be difficult to tease out what belongs where and to reach a differential formulation. It's important to clarify these possible diagnoses in order to work out the priority in terms of support for the family and therapeutic input for the child. Indeed, the severity of difficulties related to both neurodivergence and trauma will be intensified by chaotic family circumstances, frequent moves and lack of consistency and structure. Autistic children who manage their environment by 'masking', that is, suppressing their autistic traits to fit in, may be vulnerable to abuse as they attempt to conform by denying their own unique identity. Mental health professionals working in tandem with paediatricians, speech and language therapists and paediatric occupational therapists is key to meeting the needs of children with such complex presentations.

How to understand Liam? Liam was a 7-year-old boy who had shown daily extreme aggression at school coupled with sexually inappropriate behaviours. School had expressed concern that he may be autistic. Below is an excerpt from a clinic session:

Liam's play in the sand tray became free flowing, he was enjoying the sensory qualities of the sand. He increasingly played on words, e.g. 'mexicon, sandagon'. He did not seem interested in the meaning of the words but more their sounds and his ability to play with that. He appeared to have difficulty with some fine motor planning tasks such as opening and closing boxes and knowing how fragile toys were. In fact, he broke two sand toys, about which he showed no concern. When I asked about consequences, he said at school he must pay for breakages. If he breaks things at home, he has to go to jail.

Liam was referred on for an assessment for autism. Work was carried out with him on body boundaries ensuring he had the vocabulary for parts of the body and an understanding of appropriate and inappropriate touch.

It is important to understand that the treatment approaches and prognosis for children whose difficulties stem from complex trauma are different from the neurodivergent population. In the case of trauma, Music (2011, p. 95) has written about the plasticity of the brain and of the possibilities, however challenging, to affect positive change through environmental and therapeutic approaches. Whereas old experiences cannot be erased, new brain pathways can be built with new experiences. This is hopeful.

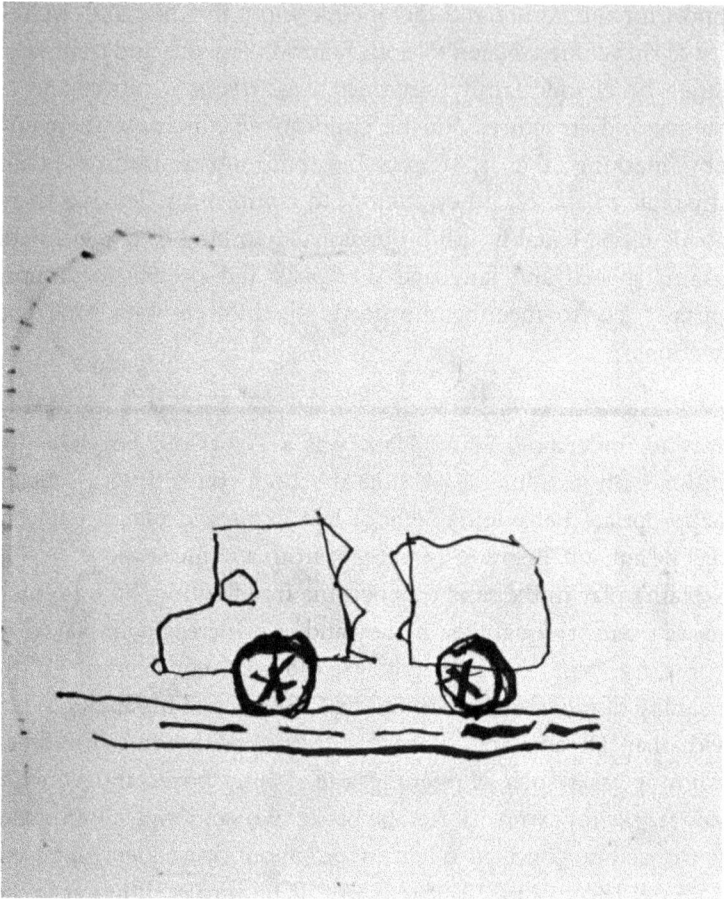

Figure 2.1 'A broken car' replica artwork based on a drawing by Liam 7 years.

Figure 2.1 shows a broken object which might represent a final rejection or a possibility of mending. There may be windows of opportunity for change particularly during the first few years of life and during adolescence when formation of new neural pathways is particularly active. The occupational therapist Sarah Lloyd has developed a model, 'BUSS', for building sensorimotor systems in children with developmental trauma (Lloyd 2020). However, autism and ADHD are lifelong conditions due to different brain organisation and cannot be made to go away or cured. Mental health support then consists of environmental adaptations, support to manage anxiety and medication when appropriate.

Reference list

BBC News. (2023). *Online News 31.01.2023*.

DSM-5. (2013). *Diagnostic and Statistical Manual of Mental Disorders*. American Psychiatric Association.

Horne, A. (2023). *A Few Reflections on Gender in Psychoanalytic Work with Children and Young People*. Notes from Intensive Study Event 10.05.2023. Human Development Scotland.

Lemma, A. (2022). *Transgender Identities: A Contemporary Introduction*. Routledge.

Lemma, A. (2023). The missing: Exploring the use of photographs in "working through" the natal body with transgender youth. *The International Journal of Psychoanalysis*, 104 (5), 809–828.

Lloyd, S. (2020). *Building Sensorimotor Systems in Children with Developmental Trauma: A Model for Practice*. Jessica Kingsley.

Melzak, S. (1999). Work with refugees from political violence. In Lanyado, M., & Horne, A. eds. *The Handbook of Child and Adolescent Psychotherapy: Psychoanalytic Approaches*. Routledge, p. 427.

Music, G. (2011). *Nurturing Natures: Attachment and Children's Emotional, Sociocultural and Brain Development*. Psychology Press.

3

PLAY AS COMMUNICATION AND AS A CHILD'S NATURAL OCCUPATION

Play is a child's natural occupation and is of central importance to the physical, emotional and social development of the growing individual. It forms the basis of much therapeutic work with children. This chapter sets out to consider what play is, why it is so important and the reasons why some children are unable to play, and adults' attitudes to children's play. Writers through the ages have explored the meaning of play and some of their thoughts will be shared in their own words throughout this section:

> Play is the highest expression of human development in childhood for it alone is the free expression of what is in a child's soul.
>
> (Froebel 1782–1852)

> For the small child play is a way of expressing his inner feelings and experiences and is as vital to his development as eating and sleeping.
>
> (Steiner 1999, p. 64)

DOI: 10.4324/9781003642862-4

> It would seem that a hunger for playfulness is inbuilt and sustains the kinds of interactions needed to build a mature human brain.
>
> (Daws and de Rementeria 2015, p. 181)

It is generally accepted that play, in contrast to working is driven by fun and pleasure. The motivation to play is intrinsic, coming spontaneously from the child, rather than involving extrinsic pressure or rewards from the child's environment. The process, rather than any achievement or end product, is central. And yet, in childhood, play is also serious business and, as in the above quote by Daws and de Rementeria (2015), one might say that there is indeed an achievement in building a mature human brain.

Play as a continuum

Babies play in order to relate to their primary carer and to explore their physical environment in relation to their own bodies. If all goes well, the way parents naturally play with their babies involves stroking, kissing, soothing, turn taking, songs and rhymes. As well as two people having fun together, such play helps the child develop both physically and emotionally (Daws & de Rementeria 2015).

The compassionate paediatrician and psychoanalyst Donald Winnicott (1971) has pointed to reciprocal interactions using eye contact and mirroring between mother and child as being at the heart of the child developing a sense of self, through being seen and held in mind by another. Through their mouths and hands and eyes babies explore shapes, textures and space: what goes in where, what happens when things are pulled or pushed, how things come apart and how they are put together again. Hearing and actual listening contributes to the baby learning how to make sounds. This is how they build a sense of their own bodies, of how things feel, of their own resources, of language, of their abilities and limitations, of what they can control and what they cannot change. Through early forms of play between parents and babies, such as the peep-boo game or throwing things away and retrieving them, children work out the boundary between me and not-me. Both these games involve practising brief separations and reunions with their care givers and can be seen as the child's way of working through anxieties about separation and abandonment in a safe way.

> The prerequisite for play is being able to hide and find, being able to bear absence because you know presence will come.
>
> (Sinason 1992, p. 186)

Toddlers continue to love playing with their parents in reciprocal ways, such as hide-and-seek, turn-taking and reading together. They enjoy their developing physical ability to manage their surroundings, climbing, running, jumping, as well as their increasing skills in building towers, stacking, throwing, tidying, drawing and using language as communication. They are careful observers and love copying adults and older children and enjoy simple pretend play. Social play at this stage consists of parallel play and sometimes handing toys to one another. Gradually, in settings with other children they learn not only about doing things but increasingly about relationships with other children, about playing together, taking turns and sharing and managing conflict and disappointment.

> Children seem to use play from a very early age as a spontaneous means of working out their relationship to the world about them, and to other people, and as a way of overcoming difficulties, whether physical or emotional.
>
> (Copley and Forryan 1997, p. 229)

Gradually, as children reach pre-school and eventually school, their play tends to involve make-believe that becomes ever more elaborate. This 'pretend play' using imagination and symbols is expanded to include suspense and excitement. Symbols can include using toys to represent a whole range of experiences in the child's world. Influences from popular culture are often woven into play themes. Alongside ongoing relationships with parents and other adults, peer friendships become important and bring joy but also require negotiation, managing conflict, broken promises and slashed wishes. Anxieties about love, hate, jealousy, pecking orders, fear of rejection and loneliness come to the fore. Some children develop their own pretend worlds and imaginary friends to help them navigate powerful emotions. Playing on the edge of fear and triumph provides children with a means of expressing and confronting their own life experiences (Hoxter 1977, p. 204).

> The purpose of play is diverse: a rehearsal for future life; dealing with anxiety and conflict; exploring the space between fantasy and reality and cognitive and social experimentation.
>
> (Horne 1999, p. 35)

In adolescence the process of separation from the primary attachment to the parents or caregivers begins. This means gradually weakening the parental bond and bringing instead influences from adolescent group culture, where the peer group in a major way can feed into a teenager's precarious and rapidly changing identity (Lanyado 1999). This happens alongside complex bodily changes, anatomical, physiological and endocrinological, and developing sexuality and gender identity. Childhood playing is replaced by teenage activities and sometimes experimentation with different forms of self-realisation. This may involve sports in teams or developing physical skills alone, playing with ideas and words, using language in line with their peer group, experimental cooking, playing music, composing, playing online and on social media. Managing the delicate balance between healthy growth and risk becomes a challenge for many young people and their parents. All such play has a need for safety and often a need for the positive interest of the care giver. During adolescence essential aspects of the personality become shaped and eventually organised into a more coherent and stable sense of self (Waddell 1998, p. 126).

Winnicott (1971) made the link between playing and cultural experience, stating that cultural experience begins with creative living. This is first manifested in play. It provides a way of seeing play on a continuum towards the development into creative experience and expression of culture in adolescence and adulthood.

> The creation of something new is not accomplished by the intellect but by the play instinct.
>
> (Jung, 2016, p. 152)

> Playing is a way of thinking. In playing, and perhaps only in playing is the individual free to be creative.
>
> (Winnicott, 1971, p. 53)

Why may some children not be able to play?

The ability for children to play and develop healthily is closely linked with the nature of early attachment relationships with parents or caregivers. Children need to have reached certain developmental milestones in order to be able to play symbolically. Their physical, cognitive and emotional development is experience dependent, meaning that the developing brain will grow differently depending on the nature and quality of care which the child receives in the earliest days, weeks and months of their lives (Music 2011). Child Psychotherapist Graham Music (2011, p. 7) states that to become a person and develop a sense of self, a child requires large amount of input from other people early in life, and an experience of ourselves as reflected back through the eyes and minds of those around us. Neglect is about the absence of such input of human contact. A child who does not have a defined sense of themselves, a sense of me-not-me in relation to their caregivers, will struggle to play in imaginative or rich ways. They cannot use make-believe either alone or with other children.

> Human connections of early reciprocal caregiving and play, shape the neural connections from which the mind emerges.
>
> (Seigal 1999, p. 2)

Children are able to play when they feel safe and held in mind by their caregivers and their external environment. They know that play is make-believe and can be interrupted should the strength of feeling become too great. In contrast, if their actual existence is threatened by violence, abuse, hunger or anxiety about the adults in their lives, preoccupation with survival takes over and spontaneous play cannot happen. The stressed and emotionally insecure child might find that their own imagination gives rise to such overwhelming anxieties that it can feel dangerous to lose themself in the play. The child needs a trusted adult to be available in mind and body to help them. That adult needs to be able to tolerate the strength of feelings expressed in the child's play without themselves becoming overwhelmed.

Without adults' emotional understanding the child might meet a blockage. The play may become chaotic, repetitive and lack coherence. Children whose play is constantly full of violence and themes of death and destruction, or inappropriate sexual behaviours, are a cause of concern and may be an indication of complex trauma (Music 2011, p. 129). Effects of adverse childhood experiences and trauma can last long after the original threat has gone and may affect children's ability to use free expression and play develop healthily into adulthood.

Children in all families experience times of feeling alone with emotions they find overwhelming. In manageable proportions, they can grow from this. However, there can be serious consequences for children who grow up neglected, and in an environment where adults are not interested in understanding them. Children who struggle to utilise play and shared play for exploration, may need additional therapeutic help.

> A child who seems unable to play is quite rightly usually a cause for concern. Play seems to be a first step in symbol formation, and thus in the ability to digest, work over and think about an important experience.
>
> (Copley and Forryan 1997, p. 229)

Adults' attitudes to playing

As we have seen, children's ability to play and to use play for exploration is closely linked with the nature of their earliest attachment relationships with the adults around them. From this follows that adults' ability to play with children and to appreciate and be respectful of children's play and playfulness may be related to their own experiences of parenting and playing.

It seems that some adults are 'naturals' at playing with children. This may take different forms. Some love the fun element of playing that may have a physical rumbustiousness about it. Others have a quieter way of engaging with children which involves curiosity and staying with what is happening in the play for the child. This curiosity may involve facilitating a child who seems to get 'stuck' or seems lost as to what to do next. Play may fluctuate between the two. When adults can be in touch with their own playfulness and creative selves they can value children's play as an important part of communication, indeed, as important as language.

For others, the ability and confidence to play with children may not come so easily and has to be learnt in a different way. This in no way means that they cannot become confident players, be they parents, teachers or therapists. Play happens in a relationship. Careful observation of young children is a helpful way to start to build up an understanding of the value of playing for the children and to value their own part in this relationship. Many parents who have missed out on rich play experiences as children struggle to give their children a space to play. Their own needs may get in the way and be expressed by the adult wanting to direct and take over. Some parents need support to feel that what they can offer their child is valuable. The mobile phone on a bus is a poor substitute to talking with their child or sharing experiences of what is happening around them. Parents may feel that they fail at play, whilst other parents are down on their knees playing trains. In fact, many types of play go unrecognised. A carer who mirrors the child's sounds as he does the household tasks, can be play. Equally, a carer who, when putting on her own socks, uses them briefly as puppets to help the child get his socks on. Parents may need help to enable playfulness to permeate their relationship with their child.

There are therapeutic parenting approaches that aim to help parents play with their child in reciprocal ways, such as Parent Infant Psychotherapy, Theraplay or Filial Therapy. All these approaches to a different extent acknowledge the need to allow a space for the parents' own needs to be recognised and addressed.

Professionals in children's services, in Child and Adolescent Mental Health Services (CAMHS) and in other clinical settings may feel that there is little space for 'just playing' in the face of expectations of 'evidence-based practice'. They may find that there is an increasing push towards standardised assessments and diagnoses. Such methods leave little space for the worker to use their own curiosity and to convey this interest to the child. Clinicians can feel that the process of playing with the child is not encouraged or valued as a valid form of assessment. And yet, with children who have suffered complex trauma, play as therapy within a firm theoretical framework often provides the only meaningful way of communicating and bringing understanding of what is going on below the surface.

A positive development in preschool and early education in Scotland is a move away from a highly directed curriculum to a more child-led approach. There is a need however to support staff in this shift towards valuing the adult-child attachment relationship as central to children's development. Child-led means encouraging staff to play with the children, respecting the children's direction of play with some guidance if need be. The concept is sometimes misunderstood to mean that children should be left to find their own way without adult help. Many children cannot manage this. They may feel lost in often large pre-school settings with limited opportunity to get to know individual staff. There is a challenge to allow staff to form relationships with the children by simply *being with them* and balance this with the requirements for early years practitioners to evidence the children's progress through paperwork and similar means.

Play and occupational therapy

Donald Winnicott in his 1971 book *Playing and Reality* provides us with a rich exploration of the development and function of play throughout the lifespan. He helps us understand the normal development of play, when it goes wrong and finally, the role of play in therapy. Winnicott's words below are equally relevant to play based occupational therapy as to psychoanalytic psychotherapy.

> Psychotherapy takes place in the overlap of two areas of playing, that of the patient and that of the therapist. Psychotherapy has to do with two people playing together. The corollary of this is that where playing is not possible then the work done by the therapist is directed towards bringing the child from a state of not being able to play into a state of being able to play'.
>
> (Winnicott 1971, p. 38)

The Italian occupational therapist Carolina de Sena Gibertoni (2013), quoted below, has translated this to her practice in her native Italy. She co-created the Vivaio model of occupational therapy which, like Winnicott, emphasises the importance of the interplay between the patient, the therapist and what she calls the 'doing'. This becomes the basis for the therapeutic relationship. This book explores how a group of UK occupational therapists found a way of putting similar ideas into practice in a CAMHS service.

> Play rules supreme in our occupational therapy rooms: children, adolescents and adults choose their activities. Motivation is an intrinsic part of choosing; it creates (with the therapist) an atmosphere of play in which anything can happen or develop. Unconscious phantasies

take up residency in events that are condensed into a real object, a movement of the body, a gesture, a scream, a song, a product that can take shape or remain unfinished. In an occupational therapy session, a piece of wood becomes a house, a ball of clay becomes a volcano.... An open, playful atmosphere allows events to unfold according to what the therapist-patient duo set in motion ....

(Gibertoni 2013, p. 43)

Reference list

Copley, B., Forryan, B. (1997). *Therapeutic Work with Children and Young People*. Cassell.

Daws, D., de Rementeria, A. (2015). *Finding Your Way with Your Baby: The Emotional Life of Parents and Babies*. Routledge.

Froebel, F. (1782–1852). Froebel trust. www.froebel.org.uk

Gibertoni, C.de S. (2013). An occupational therapy perspective on Freud, Klein and Bion. Ch 3. In Nicholls, L. et al. eds. *Psychoanalytic Thinking in Occupational Therapy*. Wiley-Blackwell, pp. 32–56.

Horne, A. (1999). Normal emotional development. Ch 3. In Lanyado, M., Horne, A. eds. *The Handbook of Child and Adolescent Psychotherapy*. Routledge, pp. 31–42.

Hoxter, S. (1977). Play and communication. In Boston, M., Daws D. eds. *The Child Psychotherapist and Problems of Young People*. Wildwood House, pp. 202–231.

Jung, C. (2016). *Psychological Types*. Routledge Classics, p. 152.

Lanyado, M. (1999). It's just an ordinary pain: Thoughts on joy and heartache in puberty and early adolescence. In Hindle, D., Smith, M.V. eds. *Personality Development*. Routledge, pp. 92–115.

Music, G. (2011). *Nurturing Natures: Attachment and Children's Emotional, Sociocultural and Brain Development*. Psychology Press.

Seigal, D.J. (1999). The developing mind: Toward a neurobiology of interpersonal experience, cited in: Balbernie, R. (2001). Circuits and circumstances: The neurobiological consequences of early relationship experiences and how they shape later behaviour. *Journal of Child Psychotherapy*, 27, 237–255.

Sinason, V. (1992). *Mental Handicap and the Human Condition*. Free Association Books, p. 186.

Steiner, D. (1999). The toddler and the wider world. In Hindle, D., Smith, M.V. eds. *Personality Development*. Routledge, pp. 48–70.

Waddell, M. (1998). *Inside Lives: Psychoanalysis and the Growth of the Personality*. Duckworth & Co.

Winnicott, D.W. (1971). *Playing and Reality*. Routledge.

4

WHAT HAPPENS IN THE PLAYROOM

In the playroom the therapist and the child need to find a way to connect emotionally. The therapy room should be a safe and containing space where together child and therapist can freely explore. The child's natural way of doing this is through play. The therapist must be aware of their own internal state, aiming to approach each session with an open mind into which the child can step.

What makes a playroom conducive to therapeutic exploration?

- predictability, so that the same room is available at the times planned
- a neutral space that the child can use in their own way
- a sand tray which is not flooded and has no toys hidden
- toys and materials that are consistent and stored so that children can see what is available

Shirley Hoxter (1977, pp. 207–208) outlines the essential equipment: 'little human figures, wild and domestic animals, cars, art materials and access to

DOI: 10.4324/9781003642862-5

water'. She explains that toys 'are there to provide the child with a vocabulary'. Elaborate play and art materials are not necessary. For adolescents the room may need to be modified to include creative arts activities and fewer young children's toys on display.

Individual therapy boxes can be used in a variety of ways. In some settings each child is given a box with their own therapy materials. A box may be the only practical way to provide a 'temporary playroom' such as in a school setting. In other settings the box can be used to hold things that the child has made or objects of special significance to the child. In each case the box is an individual confidential resource in a shared therapy room. Children often choose to individualise their boxes by decorating or colouring them. The box can be the size of a shoebox or bigger, depending on its purpose. How the contents of the box are managed can become a theme in the therapy. Should things that have broken or materials that have been used up be replenished? Can there be room for mourning what is lost and an opportunity for repair? When therapists consider whether to use boxes, then storage, resources and confidentiality need to be thought through.

Sessions take place at the same time every week and usually last 45–60 minutes. The room should be in a neutral state for the child to enter. This means that there should not be signs of previous children's play, such as scenes of miniature figures left in the sand tray or paintings by other children on display. For the room to be experienced as a safe setting for the child, it is important that interruptions are kept to an absolute minimum and that sessions start and finish on time. Many children struggle with beginnings and with endings. Indeed, the flow of the whole session becomes something to aim for over time. The therapist's management of time, space and self all contribute to a sense of containment for the entire therapeutic experience.

To get underway the child and therapist must negotiate the separation from the carer and make their journey to the therapy room. This is a significant moment to observe closely. Embedded here are patterns of attachment and ways of problem solving in the family. The therapist may need to ease the process. Parents could be encouraged to describe to the child the purpose and format of the sessions, such as 'you will be with the therapist for a while, maybe playing a game and drawing a picture and then you will come back together, and we will go home'. At times the separation is so difficult that it needs to be eased in various ways: the parent could accompany the child into the playroom and stay for a while, or the therapist and the child agree to leave the playroom after ten minutes to 'check up on Mum' before returning to the playroom for the session to continue.

Below are some case vignettes and examples of the therapist's reflections and responses, of which there are always several possibilities. These can be considered with colleagues and in supervision. Frequently the therapist may feel they have missed a moment for therapeutic intervention. However, we have found that if an urgent issue for the child has been missed by the therapist, then similar themes are likely to recur. This gives the therapist an opportunity for a different or a more considered response.

How do we observe the child's entry into the playroom?

Sometimes creative ways must be found to encourage the child to engage with the therapist.

Jane aged 5 showed sexualised behaviour towards her foster carers and teachers but had made no clear disclosures of abuse. She was referred with the request for support for the carers and teachers. Regular meetings took place, but the challenging behaviour continued. Individual assessment of Jane was agreed.

For her first appointment we met in the waiting room. Her foster father told me she had been unwilling to get out of bed this morning. I wondered how Jane would react to this implied criticism. She pretended she had not seen me. She refused to come with me yet didn't want her foster father to accompany her. I encouraged her to come, and she started stamping her way noisily out of the waiting room and up the stairs. She told me to stamp too, which I did. Our stamping became rhythmical and involved turn taking, eye contact and good humour. Our connection was beginning to form.

(Jane is referred to below and in Chapter 9)

Mirroring the child's movement in this spontaneous way marked the start of an empathic relationship. Noticing Jane's anxiety during separation from her foster father gave rise to discussions with him around appropriate expectations of a young child under stress.

How do therapists learn from the child?

What can we learn from observing the child's presentation, clothing, movement, style of separation from their carer and their understanding of attendance?

Jane (see above) was usually dressed in shorts and a T shirt. She was confident in her actions, enjoying running up and down stairs. She commented that she wasn't a girl, she was a boy and that she liked 'boy things'.

Sometimes it seemed best to repeat back to Jane that she likes 'boy things' to reassure her that she had been heard. Later in sessions the therapist was able to be more proactive in their responses, wondering aloud what things boys like. The word 'wondering' is used frequently in this text. The reason for this is that 'wondering aloud' lets the child know that the therapist is thinking about them, without any expectation of a response. Asking a direct question might put the child in a dilemma of how best to answer.

How do we orientate the child to the session?

Below are examples of some statements which the therapist might use to orientate the child to the purpose and format of sessions. One or two sentences should be used to sum up the overall purpose of sessions such as 'you'll remember your Mum told me that she thinks something is bothering you about what happened when you were living with Z'. During subsequent sessions it is likely that the child will need further issues clarified. Below are some examples of what one might say to a child at different moments:

- in this room we play, draw and think together
- I will choose what to do for the first half of your time today and you can choose what we do for the second half
- I will look after your paintings until we finish working together
- I will join in your games if you ask me to
- I will let you know if I am going to talk about our play here with anyone else
- sometimes I might not join your games because I need to think

- one of the rules here is that we keep things safe so that we both can play and think. So, we try not to break anything
- an important rule is that you are safe. So, it's against the rules to climb up onto the high windows

How do we manage boundary difficulties during early sessions?

Georgie aged 14, with a care history and an intellectual disability was referred following his allegation of sexual abuse. I walked up the stairs and into the playroom with him. That short journey was problematic. Georgie wanted to bring toys into the playroom, and he wanted to 'borrow' toys from the playroom. He liked to run around the department knocking on other clinic room doors. He threatened to jump over the bannisters.

(Georgie is also referred to below)

Boundaries about toys had to be explained to Georgie from time to time. Recognising his risky threats, he needed steering away from the bannisters. Only once he was settled in the room, it became possible to comment on his feelings and his risky responses. The therapist had to take note of his level of focus and use clear language so that he could understand. He could then be encouraged to express his emotions through play or words instead of acting them out.

How do we use materials?

Stuart aged 10, from a background of multiple foster placements and intermittent contact with his birth mother was referred with frequent angry outbursts at school and home. As part of his sessions, he usually chose to paint. This consisted of squeezing paint out of the plastic bottles directly onto the paper. During each session he would empty at least one bottle. Once the paint was on the paper, he left that activity and moved to play with the dolls' house or the cars. In this play he was involved in elaborate imaginary themes.

The emptying of paint suggested he needed to let go of some feelings before he could move into more sophisticated thinking and play. This observation was discussed with his foster carers who were able to encourage him to keep to routines so that his daily life could feel more predictable and therefore safe. Stuart's use of paint was a dilemma for the therapist. Should they allow this? Should they ensure that the empty bottles remain in the room and that eventually the paint is all used up? Should the paint be endlessly replenished?

What can we learn of the child's feelings from the content of their play?

Harry aged 8 whose mother was in poor health, set out the farm animals and told a story of how the calf got hurt. The paramedics put a fence around the calf whilst they operated on the calf. The other animals were kept out. Harry expanded the fenced enclosure little by little until the other animals were way out of sight of the calf. The calf tried to get out but couldn't and its parents tried to get in but couldn't. The calf was completely alone, surrounded by space. The other animals visited the calf but didn't know what to say, so departed.

Harry's story of the calf gave rise in the therapist, through projective identification (see Chapter 6) to feelings of loneliness and isolation. Here they remained 'in the play'. An alternative might have been to suggest that Harry might feel lonely like the calf, but this would have taken Harry's mind out of this play and the depth of his feeling might be lost or denied. In this instance, it was best to hold the feeling in mind, and 'hand it back' to Harry in a digested way at a different time. The hope was that through this recognition of the emotion, the child could feel understood.

What can we learn from the child's interaction with the therapist?

Georgie aged 14 (as in the example above) in his play gave himself the role of the boss of a dog's home. He drew a picture of himself demanding that I stick it on the wall of his office. He assigned to me the role of staff member. He told me that if anything happens, I'd have to do the first aid. However, I was forbidden to tell anyone of any accidents, because there was no insurance. There were a lot of dogs who barked and escaped. Georgie explained that a Doberman had bitten me, taking my flesh off, down to the bone. Suddenly the boss i.e. Georgie became magical/god-like. He explained that he was giving me back my skin to cover my shredded limb. In addition, he changed the weather making the snow fall, the lightning strike and the thunder boom.

The theme of Georgie's communication was sorting out danger in a magical and secret way. This implied Georgie's assumption about the lack of safety in his life. He could not turn to anyone for help and therefore had to make himself all powerful. His self-portrait suggests he has an intellectual disability (Figure 4.1).

It is poignant suggests he has an intellectual disability. It is poignant that this immature boy grabbed the role of a powerful boss, denying his sense of vulnerability. With this as a backdrop he positioned the therapist as victim and himself in control. In his story he was unable to tolerate the dreadful wounds inflicted by the dog. So, he fixed the wounds using his own omnipotence. This allowed the therapist to learn how he managed painful situations in his daily life by avoiding his own helplessness and

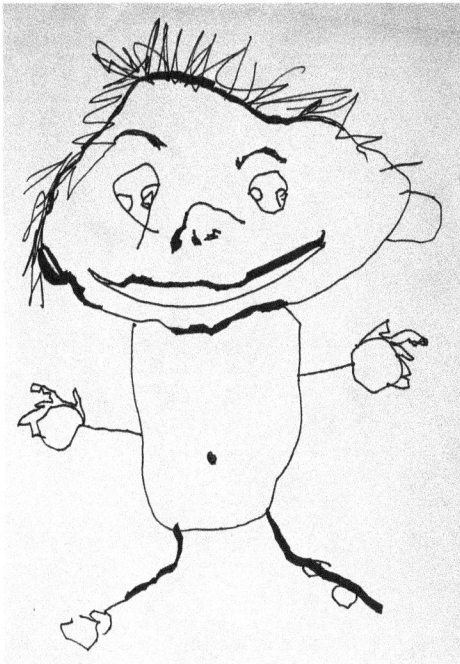

Figure 4.1 'This is me' replica artwork based on a drawing by Georgie 14 years.

using magical thinking to solve problems. The precarious weather seemed to be a further reflection of his unpredictable situation.

How do we decide whether or not to link the play with real life?

Sam aged 8 was referred by his school following the traumatic death of his aunt. He chose to make a mask of a lion. This provided the opportunity for him to try out different voices, different identities and tell several short stories. I suggested that the lion might show everyone how he can do everything and is so confident. However, I suggested that behind the mask, the lion might feel different, even maybe a bit scared. Sam avoided any such conversation, and the play remained in the metaphor.

(Sam is also referred to in Chapter 5)

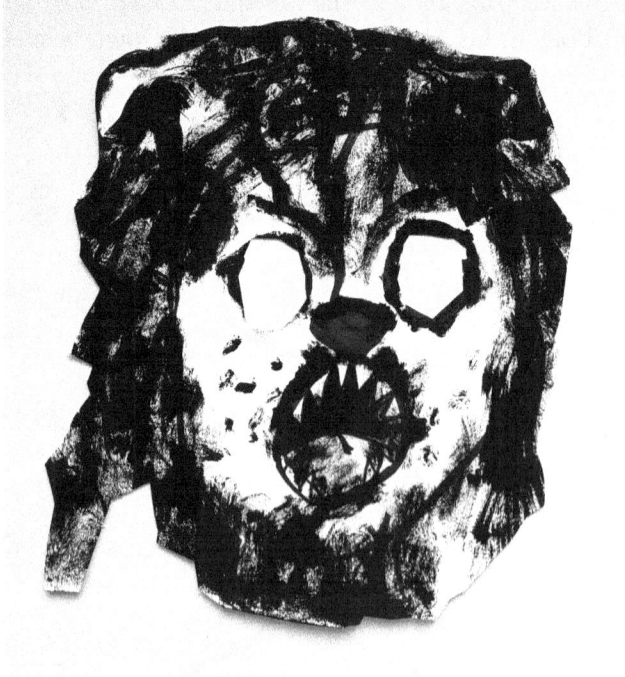

Figure 4.2 'My lion' replica artwork based on a mask made by Sam 9 years.

Sam tried hard to keep the mask up, but it was 'paper thin'.

It could be seen as a strength that Sam knew he had to keep in control, hiding disturbing emotions (Figure 4.2). The therapist needed to weigh up how much to recognise and boost his need for defences and how much to support him to peep behind them. It may have been too early to suggest that Sam was scared. In the longer term it might have indicated that Sam didn't have adequate support for engaging in therapy, and that the parents needed more support to enable Sam to 'lower his mask'.

How do we honour the child's confidentiality whilst ensuring child protection professionals are given concerning information?

Sarah aged 7 was referred with inappropriate sexual behaviour. I invited her to make a picture of everyone at home, doing things they each enjoy. I spoke little except to clarify who was who and what they were doing.

She suddenly leant down and kissed the drawing of her mother's partner 'Smiley', with whom she was not allowed contact. Her quiet focus changed, and she became alarmed and said, 'don't tell Sue (social worker), you mustn't, you mustn't!' I confirmed that I understood Sarah didn't want me to tell Sue about the kiss. I then said that I want to make sure that Sarah is looked after safely and that I would have to speak to Sue.

Sarah's need to keep secrets was clearly stated (Figure 4.3). Her picture of her family identified 'Smiley' with an 'S'. The incomplete human figures together with the cage-like structure concerned the therapist, who acknowledged the strength of Sarah's feeling but didn't promise secrecy from the social worker, with whom communication was vital. As a result, Sarah became very angry and shouted that she hated the therapist and that she would never come back. Gradually she calmed down and investigated the dolls' house.

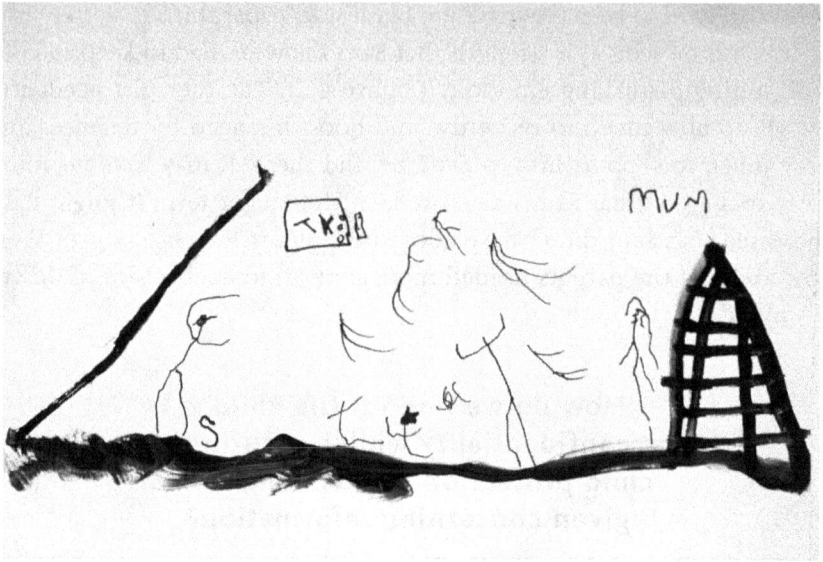

Figure 4.3 'Who is at home?' Replica artwork based on a drawing by Sarah 7 years.

How can the therapist find a helpful response in the heat of the moment?

Abu aged 12 in foster care, was referred for help with his aggressive behaviour in his foster placement and at school. He looked for the toy animals and told me that he wanted me to be a vet. He selected the lizard and taking on the lizard's voice he said, 'I want to be able to wag my tail side to side, not just up and down'. In role of vet, I asked the lizard to show me his tail wagging and suggested he try side to side wagging which he did. He was cured and went home.

Then the crocodile said, 'I want you to take out my teeth because I can't stop frightening people.' Continuing as the vet I wondered if he might be worried about his angry feelings. I told the animal that he has a good heart, and I said, 'maybe you can make your growl quieter'.

This is a complex episode of play. Abu's confusion and worry about dealing with his angry feelings were apparent. Abu brought into the play an idea that parts of himself might be able to change but he seemed to believe that the only way to make this happen was to eliminate parts of himself (his teeth). In addition, there was a suggestion of a sexual quality to Abu's play which needed to be closely monitored. In hindsight the therapist found his dilemma of anger and isolation too painful to tolerate in the moment and slipped into wanting to make him feel better.

How can the therapist be attuned to the child's pace?

Claire aged 9 was in foster care following likely sexual abuse by her father's partner. She was referred as she appeared to be confused about the abuse and why it had to stop. She painted a rainbow on a large sheet of paper. She then began to use a tiny brush to paint the sky. To complete this would take a long time.

The therapist recognised that the process of painting and thinking was of greater importance than the product. It was possible that Claire had no

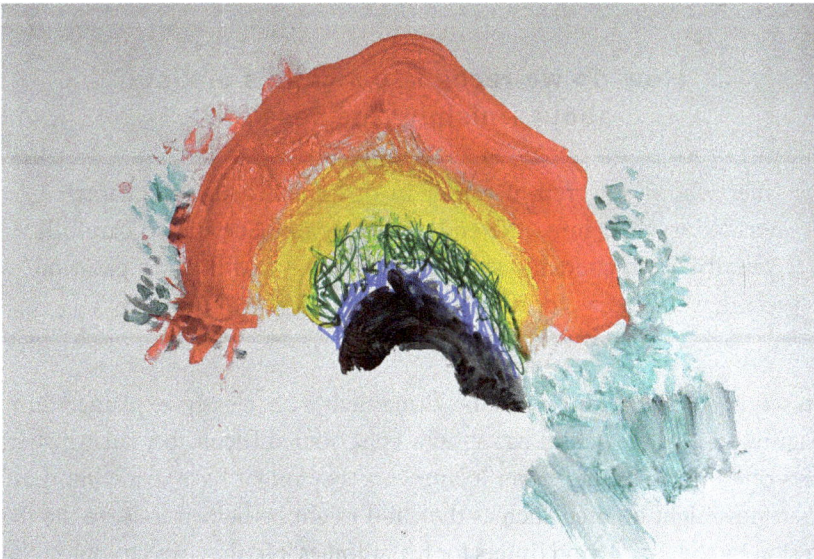

Figure 4.4 'A beautiful rainbow' replica artwork based on a painting by Claire 8 years.

wish to finish the session (Figure 4.4). Rainbows are a common theme for children and can at times be seen as defensive, only seeing the good and the beautiful.

How can we make sense of seemingly 'pointless activity'?

Leonie aged 10, in foster care due to neglect and likely factitious illness of her mother was searching through the toy boxes saying very quietly that she was looking for make-up. I then heard her say in a voice quite different from her own, 'make up is for adults'. Suddenly she changed her focus to roll and cut playdoh without making anything in particular.

The reason for this change was puzzling. Did Leonie feel a child or an adult? Did she need to distract the therapist from activities which aren't allowed? Was she anxious about her identity? The pointless quality of the play doh play left the therapist feeling Leonie's confusion.

How do we recognise a child's anxiety about finishing the session?

Jane, who is referred to earlier in this chapter and in chapter 9, decided to clear up at the end of the session. She did so carefully initially. Then suddenly she began spraying and flicking paint on to the wall, the window and my face.

This type of behaviour must be contained with clearly explained limits (Figure 4.5). After a child has shown behaviour difficult to manage, therapists often think of the 'clever' comments they might have made but didn't! Strategies might be used such as the child might be helped to leave the next session by the use of sand timers for five minutes left, then two minutes, then time to go. The child could also be given the choice of cleaning up or leaving the cleaning to the therapist. Managing the end of sessions over time was important in terms of helping Jane with transitions in general (Figure 4.6).

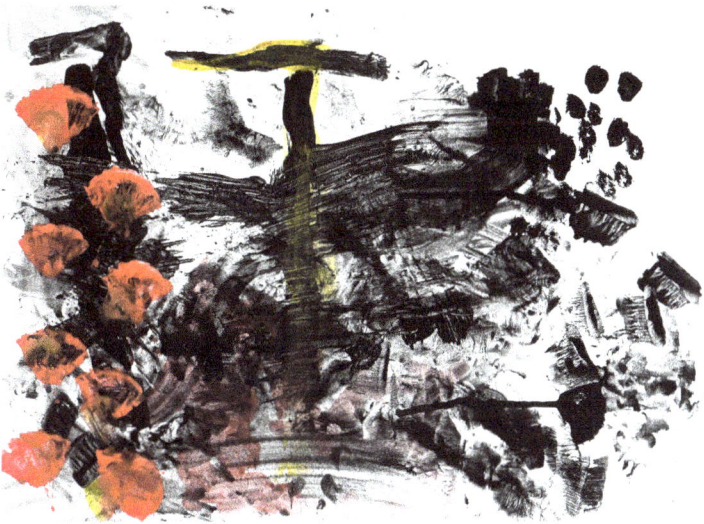

Figure 4.5 'My sad painting' replica artwork based on a painting by Jane 5 years.

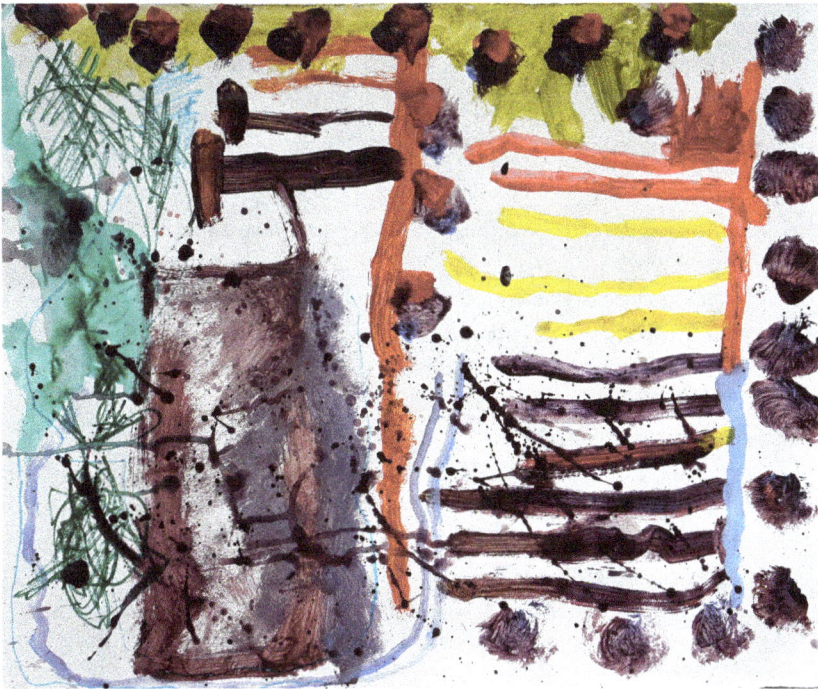

Figure 4.6 'My dance' replica artwork based on a painting by Jane 5 years.

Outside of the playroom

Therapeutic use of letters, phone and video calls

During the pandemic 2020–2022 periods of 'lockdown' meant face-to-face appointments were minimised. This formed an opportunity to try out different ways to communicate directly with children and families. Some of these ways of working have continued and been incorporated into normal practice. Initially some approaches, especially video calls, were viewed with some suspicion; however, as time went on these became part of ordinary practice.

Letters

Letters to children can take many forms. They can consist of words and/or images. They can be a single sheet of paper, or they can be a shared booklet which is sent back and forth from the therapist to the child, each adding a drawing or words. This can be a creative way of maintaining contact. Letters need to be clear in their message and appropriate for the child's developmental stage. This was one such letter which was intended to affirm Jennifer's (aged 12) use of sessions and to provide a format for her to think about the work undertaken and to offer a plan.

> Dear Jennifer
> Now that your therapy has finished, I want to tell you that you did some really good work in your therapy appointments. When we started sessions back in January, it was difficult to speak about things which had happened to you. It was difficult to play. You felt constantly scared. We made those towns in the sand tray where all sorts of things happened. Some were scary things, others were funny. You made all those stories and together we thought about them. We wondered how the children felt, especially going into the school after the confusing things happened.
>
> We talked about how when something bad has finished happening, our brains still go on expecting that bad stuff to continue. At those moments you described feeling trembly and sick.
>
> Gradually you found it easier to play and to think about the stories which happened in the sand.

Last week you felt you had done enough for the moment. You wanted to get on with schoolwork. So together we reviewed your progress.

The scared feelings had stopped. You found it much easier to get to sleep.

You can show this letter to Y at your school if you like. I will send a copy of it to your GP and to P, your social worker as they are looking out for you.

Sometimes children like to take a break and then come back here after a gap. If you would like to do that then please tell your foster carers and phone this number 8 788 7787 so we can arrange an appointment time.

You have done some courageous work Jennifer

Best wishes

Phone calls

When working with children in care it is unfortunately not unusual for a child to move unexpectedly, maybe geographically distanced from the existing services. It is important that endings are clearly understood by the child and that the therapist can be present to acknowledge their feelings.

Following one year of regular sessions with Evie aged 7, there was a sudden breakdown in her foster placement. She was moved to live in a small residential unit 40 miles away. Because of the circumstances I had not had the opportunity to say goodbye to her. To help her with the transition, I arranged with the unit for weekly phone calls with Evie.

For the first few weeks Evie told me about her new surroundings, her activities and her bedroom. She was humorous about the pets. She appeared to enjoy our dialogue. Given the richness of our previous face to face sessions this contact felt to me shallow and I questioned its value. Nonetheless by keeping in touch, it seemed to me to be honouring her memories and history. It made it easier for her to remember and refer to some of her past whilst she settled into the next phase of her life.

By the second month of phone calls Evie was having difficulty both continuing the phone calls and ending the phone calls. Her chosen subject matter became mainly her new relationships and new school. She no longer mentioned her previous carers or school and I felt that Evie's past was slipping away. Previous 'anchor points' disappeared, and Evie became disorientated if I referred to her history. Although it may have seemed she was denying the pain around loss of previous relationships, the fact that she could tell me about her new life could also be seen as a healthy readjustment and an indication that she was settling into her new environment. I suggested we had two more phone calls. These were very brief.

Video calls

During lockdown, video calls with young children were most successful if the child lived in a settled environment with parents who were able to facilitate this type of contact. They needed to be involved in setting up the technology necessary at the right time and in a quiet calm area of the house. Once set up, the parents would leave the child safely in their therapy space. The parent could of course be called if needed, otherwise the session was private. Video calls were only used for child-led play if such work had already begun in person and a good relationship with the therapist and the family had been formed. Each child had a box of toys and drawing equipment provided by Child and Adolescent Mental Health Services, kept at the child's home to be solely for use in the sessions.

Zoe aged 9, who had been sexually abused by a teacher, responded well to video sessions. Her parent set her up on a low table with drawing equipment. At each session she drew pictures and told stories. These provided an opportunity to address her turmoil.

In contrast, Hamish aged 6, was developmentally too young to be able to manage the transfer from face-to-face sessions to the use of video calls.

His mother had set him up with the computer on his top bunk bed. Hamish placed the toys on the edge of his bed so that one by one they fell to the floor. His speech was unclear though it appeared he was describing a scene of disaster. He repeatedly climbed down to get the toys, not showing any interest in whether I could see him or his play. It seemed that he was developmentally too young to grasp two-way communication over a screen.

Rory aged 7 (see Chapter 7) had been in long-term weekly therapy when lockdown occurred. He had fortnightly video sessions to maintain contact in the hope of restarting face to face therapy as soon as possible.

'I'm just getting something!' Rory went off screen and returned with a soft toy frog who started to jump making a squeaky baby sound. I asked if he wanted me to get my frog. He looked up and said, 'yes, please'.

Rory made his frog jump, and I copied him. Thus, the two frogs started jumping together. I felt it affirming that such reciprocal play could happen on screen.

As would be expected, video calls were more successful with older children. Whatever the method of non-face-to-face contact, certain parameters were essential: time, place and privacy.

Reference list

Hoxter, S. (1977). Play and communication. In Boston, M., Daws D. eds. *The Child Psychotherapist and Problems of Young People*. Wildwood House, pp. 202–231.

5

ASSESSMENT, REVIEW AND PLANNING

For which children is play based occupational therapy most appropriate?

Whilst many children with whom we work would benefit from the experience of child-led engagement we recognise that individual therapeutic play can be a scarce resource in these days of high referral rates. Nonetheless, the richness of this intervention provides valuable assessment and information and thus can be economic in terms of quality and identifying pathways for future interventions.

The target group are carefully selected vulnerable children with complex needs or those with a history of complex trauma. Many of these children are care experienced with multiple disrupted placements and significant attachment difficulties. These children are hard to reach. They are unlikely to engage with a more direct approach or with 'talking therapy'. They are at significant risk of developing mental health disorders in adulthood.

DOI: 10.4324/9781003642862-6

Assessment

Within our Child and Adolescent Health Service (CAMHS) a child may be referred specifically for play based occupational therapy because of a history of complex trauma. Some referrals are received from a member of the multi-disciplinary team for a particular assessment. This may be to gain an understanding of the child's patterns of attachment, insight into their internal world or their understanding of a specific event or experience in their life. It may have been difficult to engage a child with more standard talking interventions. An initial meeting is arranged with parents/carers and any other relevant agencies involved, often social work. This meeting enables information gathering of the child's developmental history, presenting problems and to identify aims and expectations of the assessment. This is followed by three to six sessions with the child. A review meeting is arranged with the parents and professionals, to discuss the outcome and make recommendations.

The focus of play based assessment of the child includes their

- emotional and developmental stage
- capacity to recognise, reflect and manage their feelings
- communication, attachment and relationship styles
- worries and preoccupations

It is an opportunity for the therapist to

- build an initial picture of the child's internal world
- build a relationship with the child through play and observation
- where appropriate, contribute relevant information to support the wider formulation and diagnoses

Alison aged 5 was referred with sexualised behaviour following experiences of being present when adult sexual activity took place. She lived with parents who were both addicted to street drugs. Following work with parents Alison commenced therapeutic assessment. During the first few sessions Alison insisted that she paint a grid and that we play noughts and crosses. She needed help to create a grid but was unable to ask. The game became chaotic, and Alison became irritable, sighing and spitting. When painting she resisted my suggestion that she wear an apron and refused my offer of help with the tie, twisting and writhing to both come close to me and pull away. During this she laughed, yet to me it didn't seem funny.

The therapist noted

- Alison's need to be in control
- her difficulty asking for help
- her confusion about who can keep her safe
- her sexualised writhing mixed with her ambivalence about contact with adults
- her difficulty with feelings of trust

These observations contributed to ongoing multi agency work with parents.

We describe in Chapter 4, 'What happens in the playroom' how these sessions are set up and many of the issues that frequently arise. The referral should contain information about the child's history and the current concerns. Although this information will have been shared at the initial adults' meeting, it is helpful to first meet the child with an open mind, free of assumptions. Bion (1967) wrote that the therapist should 'listen without memory or desire' (Symington & Symington, 1996). The assessment is about gathering information from the experience of being with the child, what happens in the relationship and within the play.

During the course of the assessment sessions, and indeed at different times in ongoing long-term work, the therapist will experience a lack of certainty or understanding of the child's communication and play. Tolerating 'not-knowing' what is happening within the relationship is indeed an important component of therapy, a state of mind the child needs the therapist to experience, perhaps reflecting the child's own state of confusion or defence from painful thought (Lanyado and Horne 1999).

> The build-up includes what may be lengthy periods of the therapist containing painful feelings and thoughts projected onto them by the patient, without understanding what they are about.
>
> (p. 66)

Lanyado and Horne go on to suggest that premature 'knowing' or interpretation will not be helpful.

The playing out of scenes of violence is one of the many themes that can leave the therapist 'not knowing'. Scenarios that involve guns, interpersonal violence and destructive events are not uncommon and it is likely they are on the increase as more children are exposed to inappropriate video games, TV and access to the internet. This does not necessarily mean that there is violence in the home, but allowing the themes to play out, containing feelings evoked, observing, reflecting, keeping an open mind and considering the contexts will facilitate the emergence of fuller understanding of meaning.

Assessment activities structured by the therapist

While the sessions will be largely child-led, the therapist may introduce structured tasks for the purpose of assessment:

- drawing with a specific subject, for example, my family or my island
- structured story telling using selected toy figures or animals. The therapist can start a story, and the child can take it from there to make it their own
- making three wishes

Drawing with a specific subject
My family

This is an adaptable activity. Different instructions might be: 'Draw everyone at home', 'Paint your family doing what they like doing'. Different lengths of time can be allocated to this activity and a variety of materials used. Some children need more encouragement than others, especially if they are anxious about drawing. The therapist needs to be mindful that the notions of 'family' or 'home' may have difficult associations. This is especially the case for care experienced children. Throughout this activity the therapist accepts the child's choices. Family members may be missed out, dead friends might be included, pets may be included even if they only exist in the child's mind (Figure 5.1).

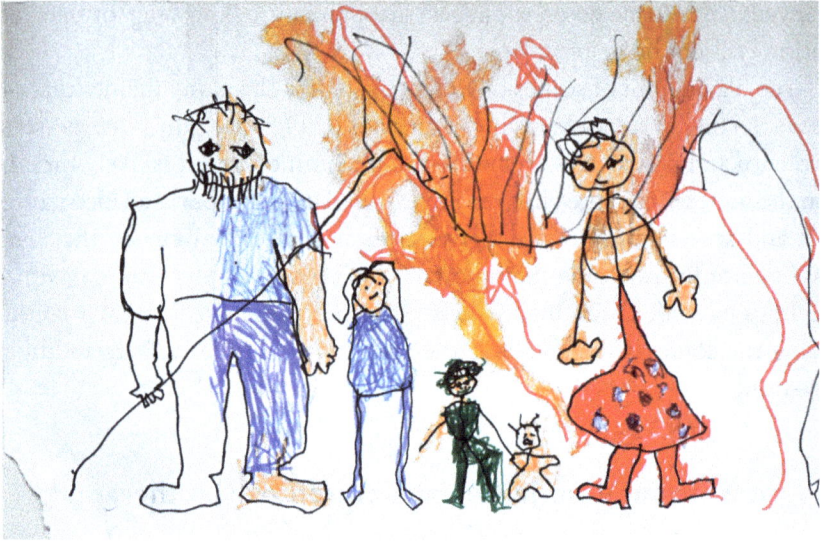

Figure 5.1 'My family' replica artwork based on a painting by Sam 9 years.

Sam, who was referred following the death of his aunt, drew his family lined up, well dressed, and carefully coloured. In contrast, behind the family Sam drew a massive, erupting volcano. Sam pointed out that the lava was about to engulf his family.

(Sam is also referred to in Chapter 4)

There is a stark contrast here between the apparent order of the family against a background of looming danger. In this threatening context, there was a sense that Sam was trying to maintain 'normality' in the family.

My island

Instructions to the child could be, 'draw/paint an island. You can make it just as you want'. 'You can choose some people or animals who you would like there and some things to play with'. 'You could think about what food you might choose'.

James aged 11, was referred following sexual abuse by his uncle against a background of his mother's chronic illness. James's island was painted very carefully. He paid particular attention to a boat, painting life jackets, a motor, oars and a sail. The boat had a first aid kit on board. Whilst the sky was clear blue, there was a grey cloud with rain falling which he explained was coming to the island. Two beds were on the sand under parasols, one with a figure asleep who he told me was his mother. His T shirt and shorts were hanging on a tree drying from a swim.

James explained his image as he painted and brought many themes to the fore. In particular he was interested in safety and possible ways to leave the island. Most of the paper was left empty. Different elements of this image and the way he painted it were discussed at the time and became useful to refer back to later in therapy.

Three wishes

Asking the child about their three magic wishes can be a way of accessing a child's dreams and fantasies and tune into their inner world. How does the child think of their wishes? Spontaneously, thoughtfully or in a laboured fashion? Can the child allow themselves to 'waste' their wishes on something frivolous? What of the child who has no wishes? Have they given up all hope, are they not able to risk thinking of good things for fear of being let down? Is their sense of self so fragile that they cannot think? Are their wishes child-like, magical or suggesting a child who carries the weight of the world on their shoulders? How do they prioritise what is important to them?

Kate aged 9 was a child with a physical disability who had to undergo numerous painful operations and walked supported by a walking stick. Her family and hospital clinicians had become increasing concerned that Kate was not coping well with this, that she was sad and upset and angry to the extent that she was attacking others with her stick. In the initial session with Kate,

I asked her what her three magic wishes might be. She immediately answered:

1. That her dad would not be away for such long stretches at a time
2. That her mum and dad would get along better
3. That her big brother would be nicer to her

I wondered aloud with Kate how it was that, even though the reason that she came to see me had been to do with her leg, her wishes were not about that. They turned out to be about her family. She looked at me intently and said, 'my leg would have been my fourth wish'.

This changed our initial formulation, and we were able to continue our clinical contact working with the family rather than with Kate individually.

Some children have difficulty imagining how anything could be different/better than what they know now (Figure 5.2).

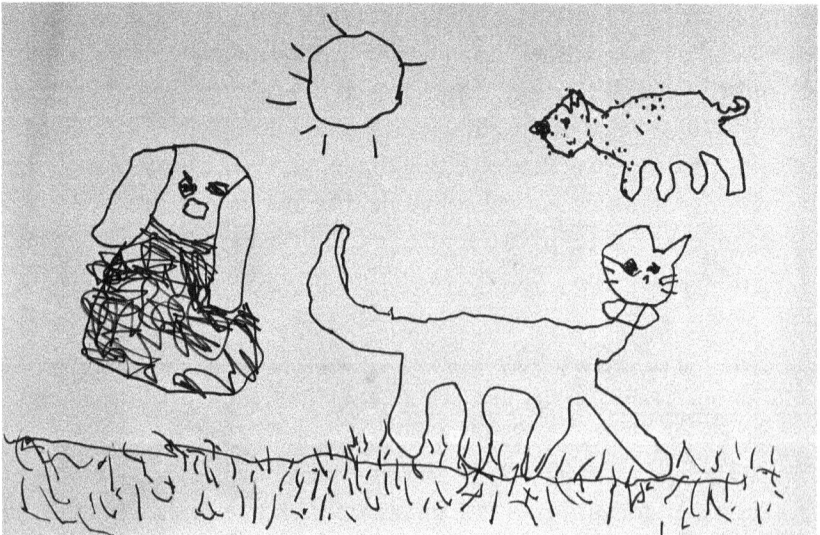

Figure 5.2 'My three wishes' replica artwork based on a drawing by Amy 9 years.

Amy, aged 9, referred for support with school refusal against a background of maternal intellectual disability, was asked for three things she wished for. Amy looked at me with a puzzled expression. Only with encouragement did she manage to say she wants a dog and a rabbit.

Then she said she is getting a cat. Already I was muddled but I reminded her about the third wish. She said, 'I want to paint the walls of my room blue'. Then she said she likes pink.

Surprisingly she said, 'It is pink already.' I felt Amy's confusion and difficulty. I commented how difficult it can be to think what could be different.

Amy's response reflected her difficulty with the task. It was also difficult for her to know who was responsible at home for making changes.

Alongside what happens in the playroom and before the review, the remit of a play based assessment is also to gather information about the child from a variety of sources – family, school, social work and any other relevant agencies. A good developmental history will be useful but not always easy to get, perhaps requiring reference to social work and community child health records. These children often have complex histories which may have spanned different geographical areas and agencies and information may not have been consistently shared. For children who have experienced neglect, a direct consequence is that significant medical conditions can go undiagnosed and therefore untreated for years. Examples of this would be partial sightedness, deafness and significant speech or dental problems. Medical conditions caused by parental addiction to drugs and alcohol such as foetal alcohol syndrome can make children hard to care for and may be hard to diagnose.

This again underlines the importance of interagency communication and working.

Review

When setting up dates for the child's sessions, our practice has been to also arrange a date for a review with professionals, the relevant adults and perhaps the child. The purpose is to give feedback, to make sense of the sessions within the context of the child's history, development and relationships, and to agree on a way forward. In the last play session, we would remind the child which adults will be attending the review meeting, what might be talked about and what feedback we plan to give about their sessions. We would ask for their permission on the feedback and ask what they thought about the sessions. It may be that older children would want to be present but there may also be meetings where delicate discussions are expected, and their attendance for only a short part of the meeting would be a desirable.

The issue of confidentiality can also be tricky. We will have explained at the beginning of sessions that what we do together in the playroom is private, but also that our job is about keeping the child safe and if we are ever worried about that safety, we might have to speak to someone else who could help (i.e., we will explain Child Protection in very simple way). We will have said that we will let them know before we have to do that. However, when it comes to the review meeting, a balance must be considered about how much of the child's communication to the therapist should be shared. Putting aside the obvious question of any child protection issues, the sessions need to be made meaningful but not exposed in a way that is emotive or disrespectful. Discussing the themes of play with parents is often the best way to do this. The therapist can make a tentative explanation of the meaning of the child's play. This would be based on their experience of being with the child, knowing the context, their theoretical understanding and their clinical judgement.

Making child-led play meaningful to others can be challenging and requires the therapist to be sensitive to the audience, particularly with parents, around issues which could be construed as judgemental of their parenting or blaming. It may be that some of the material that the child has communicated has been disturbing and will be difficult for parents to hear. However, it will often be a relief for parents to have confirmation of their concerns about the child. It may be helpful to remind the meeting that you will follow up with a written report to give everyone a chance to digest what has been covered.

The task for the therapist when giving feedback is to provide a formulation of the child's development and current difficulties through a trauma and attachment framework. Recommendations should be discussed regarding a way forward. It is important to find out what those adults involved think about the feedback and the plans. All of the above, covered during the review meeting, should then be incorporated into what can become a fairly lengthy formal report. Of course, reviews should also be held at regular intervals during the course of ongoing long-term therapy.

Planning

Following the assessment, recommendations can be made. Within CAMHS there are a number of possibilities of the best way forward, which include

- continued play based therapy. This is an option when the child wishes to continue, their care circumstances are reasonably stable, the parents are motivated and can commit to bringing the child to sessions as well as support any potential fallout from difficult issues arising in sessions
- continued direct work with the child building foundation skills such as emotional or stress regulation skills. These would form a vital step before trauma processing or other trauma focused therapy
- parenting support for the parents with a focus on attachment and secondary trauma, that is, the effects of living with child experiencing trauma
- consultation to the system
- referral for specialist assessment, for example, attachment styles, neurodivergence, maybe with other members of the multidisciplinary team

It has been our experience at CAMHS, that children with very complex presentations often benefit from a staged approach with different treatments at different times. This could be a period of play based therapy followed by more direct trauma focused work, or other variations, sometimes introducing a new therapist with a new approach, sometimes staying with the original relationship. Children's circumstances change. The child's development brings new priorities. It would be easy to consider that all these vulnerable patients would benefit from the consistent approach we can offer in long term child-led therapy. We need always to consider what can be most helpful at each stage of the child's development.

The following case study of Chloe gives a summary of how individual assessment sessions were shared with the system around her and resulted in further work with the carers, rather than Chloe alone.

CHLOE

Chloe was a six-year-old girl who was removed from her birth parents when aged 3 because of neglect, parental drug and alcohol misuse and domestic violence. Chloe experienced three previous care placements and was in permanent foster care at the time of the therapy. She presented as a girl with developmental trauma, disorganised attachment and developmental delay.

BEGINNING

Session 1 – In the waiting room, Chloe and her female carer who she called Mum, were busy with a puzzle. She introduced me to Chloe, and I was surprised at the speed with which she separated from her. Chloe walked up the corridor ahead of me even though she had never been in the building before. She did not know what room we would use and had never met me. I noticed her slightly stiff and awkward gait and the words 'brave little soldier' came to mind as if she was stealing herself for a bit of an ordeal.

In the playroom I asked her if she wanted to take off her coat because it was warm, but she refused. She was quick to look around, taking in the room and toys, but paying little attention to me, as I explained simply what we would be doing over the 6 sessions, a little of what I knew about her and who I would be talking to about our play together. I was aware of being very careful with my words, conscious of her anxiety and realising that she was not taking much in.

She moved around the room as if she were memorising where things were rather than taking an interest in what they were. This lasted for a few minutes. I stayed seated and occasionally commenting on what she was looking at and wondering aloud if she was working out what the room was about and what she might want to do.

She took the lid off the sandpit, and I brought over two little chairs so that we could sit together. She put her hands in the sand and rummaged about without any sense of what next, so I suggested she could put animals or people or anything from the toy trays into the sand to make a story. She chose some figures and buried them in the sand. While I talked quietly to her and asked a few questions like what she liked to play with at home and what the names of her cats were, she answered me and gave me sidelong glances. Her voice was very quiet and her speech was difficult for me to understand. I was reminded of the very many developmental challenges she was facing.

This sort of activity was repeated two or three times with her starting to look at some of the toys, but nothing seemed to hold any real interest for her. When I suggested drawing, she relaxed into that a little more and produced a number of quick pictures - a football, a cat, a car. I asked her if she could draw me a picture of her family and she agreed. A number of figures emerged drawn over several different pieces of paper and I noticed that she seemed unaware of the edges of the sheets of paper in front of her, so that the process became a bit chaotic. She explained that she had drawn her foster mum (a large figure) and dad, her two foster sisters and their two cats. She then drew herself as a little figure in the same group although across different sheets, and an even smaller baby figure called Katie. Katie was her sister and when I asked her if she lived in their house, she said she wasn't sure

Therapist's reflection

I was aware just how anxious Chloe was in this first session and how difficult it was for her settle to play. She needed to familiarise herself with the space before she could feel safe. It made me think of the number of moves she had experienced and how precarious her sense of permanence and containment was. I suspected that her level of anxiety hugely

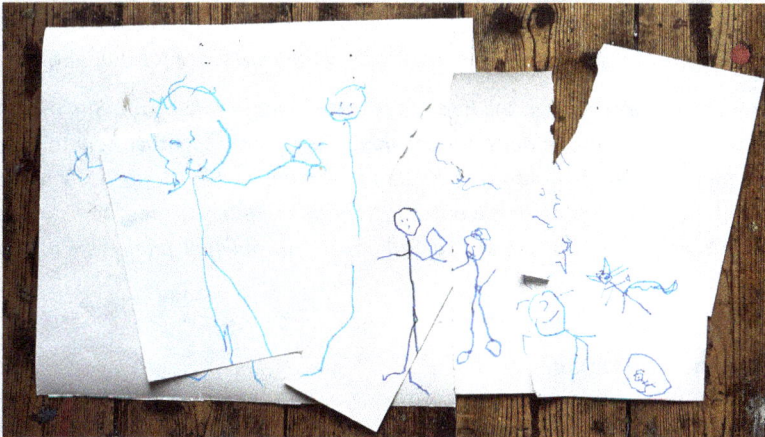

Figure 5.3 'Family' replica artwork based on a drawing by Chloe 6 years.

influenced her physical and cognitive abilities so that I was seeing Chloe operating from a younger stage. I also wondered about the fragmented way she portrayed her family and her confusion about where her sister Katie lived (Figure 5.3).

MIDDLE

Session 4 - Chloe immediately commented on toys in the room which she recognised were not in the same place as last week. She repeated the question for several items that I had not noticed, in my haste, were out of their usual place. She seemed to accept my reflection that she had wanted everything to be just the same and my apology that I hadn't managed to make it right for her.

There then followed a long sequence of activity where she systematically moved all the toys, boxes, furniture, shifting everything back flat against the walls - turning, pulling, pushing, repositioning everything with great physical effort and determination. Objects were stacked on top of each other, with emphasis on squeezing and squashing smaller things under the structures that she made with the bigger furniture. She asked for no help and ignored me when I offered. She made no eye contact and no conversation. I reflected on how busy she was, how important it felt that she put everything in the right place and that she will do it all herself. I wondered if she needed it to feel tidy and in order. I wondered if things were safer tucked underneath other things, and she surprised me by commenting that she used to do that. The activity felt full of anxiety and compulsion, with little space for thought.

At last the storm passed, she had made the playroom safe again. She moved on to some play in the dolls' house where we explored together how to keep the roof from leaking onto the children in the house. She dripped the water out of the baby feeding bottle onto the roof and wanted the roof to be made watertight with bits of paper and Sellotape. This play felt finally like a joint endeavour.

Therapist's reflection

I remember this first 30-minute section of Chloe's session as being highly uncomfortable. I had been immediately confronted with my mistake by not ensuring continuity in the playroom, particularly given Chloe's history. I felt careless, another neglectful adult, not meeting her needs.

The almost manic activity was very painful to witness – I felt useless to her, shut out, unable to help with her heroic efforts to feel safe and in control. I wondered about intervening in a more directive way, but this activity felt like something she needed to communicate without interruption. I wondered silently about her experience of protecting her baby sister, perhaps sheltering them both from the crashing, angry giants of her early days or from the unsafe and leaky roof.

ENDING

Session 6 I reminded Chloe that this was to be the last session for now, and I explained how the grown-ups would have a meeting to decide what we thought would be helpful for her. I asked her what she thought about coming to play with me and she fixed me with her slightly puzzled sideways gaze as if wondering what she should say. Quickly, without answering, she started to move around the edges of the room checking the placement of the toys and furniture. She settled in front of the dolls' house, but this held her attention for only a few moments and then she asked to do some drawing.

She wanted to join pages together and tried to manipulate the Sellotape and scissors. She accepted my helping with the task and then after a few minutes became very animated and demanded that I stick the tape up onto the wall. There followed a long piece of play during which she directed me to attach tape high up on the wall and then stretch it over to the opposite wall. Then I was to stretch more tape across the other walls so that they crossed over in the centre. This was no easy task as it demanded of me a lot of clambering about on furniture to reach the height she wanted, and technical frustrations as the tape peeled itself away from the wall. Once the lines were joining the walls and crossing over each other, she wanted pieces of paper on which she had made some scribbles, to be stuck to the lines. She was very much in charge of the action in a way that was confident and in control. She laughed when I commented that they looked like washing on a line.

It was time for us to finish, and Chloe declared that it was time for her to cut the tapes. Climbing up on a chair she struggled with the scissors, making several attempts which eventually were successful. Despite my anxiety about her feeling upset when they were cut, she managed, and returned to her mum, throwing herself into her lap.

Therapist's reflection

I was aware of how different this session had felt with Chloe very much in control, and of how important the 'taping' of her space had been to her. I felt that familiar sense of not being sure what had just taken place. I had been working hard to make it right for her, feeling concern when the tapes slipped, or about how she would respond when the tapes were cut even though she had been in control of their destruction. How would she tolerate the cutting of these 'ties'? Chloe had experienced so many shattering endings – was she taking charge of this one? Returning to the playroom after she had left the department, to the tangle of tape and paper, I was struck just how much she had made her mark on the room, and on me.

Assessment review and treatment plan

After Chloe's six sessions, I met with her carers and the two social workers involved, to give them some feedback and make plans going forward. I learned that there were a couple of additional changes in Chloe's life – her much loved teacher had gone off on long-term sick leave, and there was an acceleration of the plan to have her little sister Katie come to live in the family (visits and overnights were becoming more frequent). The carers had felt that she had found the sessions difficult, was very tired afterwards and not able to return to school for the afternoon. Generally, at home Chloe had been very unsettled, sleeping badly, much more agitated and seemed to have taken a step back with some of her developmental gains. It was interesting to learn that while she had said very little to me about her birth family or the very many losses and traumas she had experienced, she had made a couple of comments to her carers. She had also begun to talk about how her head and body felt when she was scared.

I fed back about our sessions together, covering a number of aspects to her presentation – her high level of anxiety and its impact on many aspect of function (overactivity, speech, cognition), a lack of coherent narrative to her life story, her fragile attachment system and need for physical safety, that she had begun to bring trauma memories to sessions but was not yet able to tolerate direct reflection, a sense of responsibility for keeping her baby sister safe.

As a group we were able to discuss how this kind of work can destabilise children, particularly if their emotional regulation skills are immature, as was the case for Chloe. She had several big changes happening in the external world. Her carers were clearly cautious about continuing exploratory work at this stage and I agreed that it would be helpful for Chloe to have stronger foundations before we continued with trauma processing.

This can often be the outcome of a play based assessment. The timing may not be right for ongoing child-led sessions and a staged approach may recommend other more directed input at that point in the child's development, or because of their particular situation. In Chloe's case we set up sessions with her and her carer attending together, to do some very basic anxiety management, supporting Chloe to understand the strange bodily sensations she had become aware of and have some strategies to help. Sessions became a time when Chloe was able to tolerate explanations of what the plans were for her sister's care, and other unsettling events. A little further down the line, her carer and I put together a narrative, in the third person, with details close enough but not so close, that brought together several aspects of Chloe's early disjointed experiences into a cohesive story. She would ask for this to be read to her in sessions and took it home to share with her family. I was reminded of Chloe's earlier attempts to join up the room with tape, with its hanging disjointed words.

Reference list

Lanyado, M., Horne, A. (1999). The therapeutic relationship and process. In Lanyado, M., Horne, A. eds. *The Handbook of Child and Adolescent Psychotherapy: Psychoanalytic Approaches*. Routledge, pp. 55–72.

Symington, J., & Symington, N. (1996). *The Clinical Thinking of Wilfred Bion*. Routledge, pp. 166–174.

6

THEORETICAL UNDERPINNING OF PLAY BASED OCCUPATIONAL THERAPY

As therapists we need an understanding of both individual and systemic factors that contribute to the difficulties faced by our child clients and, furthermore, how these factors can affect therapeutic relationships and the choice of interventions. The theoretical foundation may vary from therapist to therapist and will depend on level of experience, nature and extent of any postgraduate training, individual interests and the theoretical leanings of close colleagues and supervisors. It is helpful to see our theory base as a dynamic underpinning for our work, which can be questioned and adapted over time as we learn from experience.

A firm theoretical base

- guides the therapist in their doing/playing with the child
- helps the therapist hypothesise about a case at referral stage, even before direct contact, and to decide on possible ways forward
- can help the therapist make sense of what happens in the therapy room with the child and to reach a workable formulation

DOI: 10.4324/9781003642862-7

- helps the therapist communicate their assessment with families and fellow professionals
- can protect therapists from becoming overidentified with one part of the system so that they remain able to see all the factors impacting the child
- prevents the therapist being sucked into the prevailing dynamics of the case which would risk those being re-enacted rather than reflected upon
- provides a framework for the therapist that allows the therapeutic work to be held safely within professional and ethical boundaries

We begin with a discussion about the importance of clinical observation as a basis for play based occupational therapy (PBOT). This includes an exploration of what it means to develop observational skills. The importance of a child's early experiences is discussed.

We then describe theoretical concepts that overlap and form an integral part of our practice and without which this work could not take place. We cover relevant neuroscience, psychoanalytic and related theories and systemic issues that impact on individual therapy with children. We follow

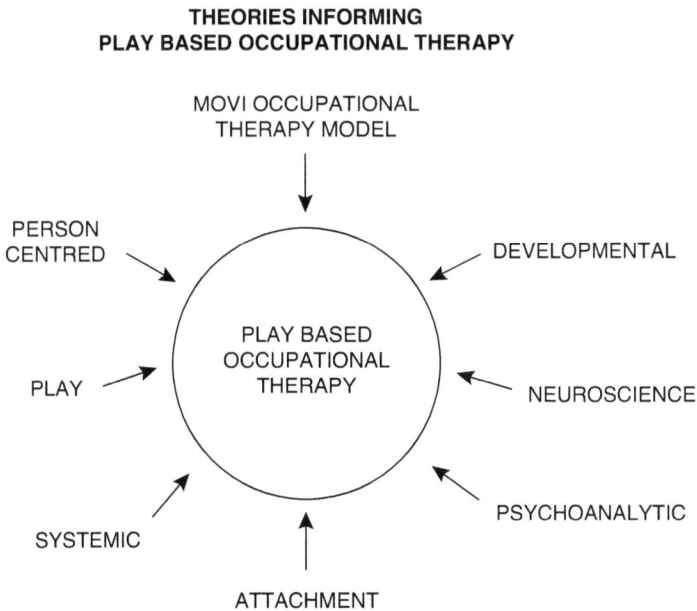

THEORIES INFORMING
PLAY BASED OCCUPATIONAL THERAPY

MOVI OCCUPATIONAL
THERAPY MODEL

PERSON
CENTRED

DEVELOPMENTAL

PLAY BASED
OCCUPATIONAL
THERAPY

PLAY

NEUROSCIENCE

SYSTEMIC

PSYCHOANALYTIC

ATTACHMENT

Figure 6.1 Theories informing play based occupational therapy.

this with a section on the practice model of Vivaio model (MOVI) of occupational therapy as a useful occupational therapy framework. We end this chapter with a reminder of the principles of person-centred, non-directive therapy, which continue to be helpful when forming therapeutic relationships with children (Figure 6.1).

Developing a psychodynamic observational stance

In play based occupational therapy, we simultaneously observe, reflect and decide how to respond. Afterwards, writing up sessions, during supervision or with colleagues, we reflect some more. Good observational skills are at the core of such reflecting, which of course then leads to good assessment.

Therapists working in Child and Adolescent Mental Health Services (CAMHS) have found it useful to undertake further training in developing their therapeutic skills through the systematic observation of infants and young children. This usually involves regular observation of an infant in their home environment and the opportunity to discuss the detailed recordings in a supportive setting with the seminar group. Such training was originally devised by Esther Bick and has long formed an integral part of the training of child psychotherapists and other professionals undertaking courses in therapeutic skills with children (Bick 1964). Such observation and subsequent sharing of reflections in a seminar group gives an intimate insight into early emotional development and attachment relationships. It also helps the observer develop an observational stance and be aware of their own countertransference (see below) reactions. The observer actively experiences what is going on but is not able to intervene in any way.

Baby observation when baby Sophie was six weeks old, at home with her mum Michelle and her sister Eliza, aged 3½:

Michelle opened the door with Eliza in tow. From the living room an intense baby cry could be heard. As I entered, I saw Sophie half lying, leaning on a cushion in a chair. As we came in her crying stopped and she seemed asleep. Eliza and I sat down, and Michelle left the room. For about 5 minutes Sophie seemed peaceful in the chair with her eyes closed. Eliza showed me her baby doll, pointing to Sophie, saying 'my baby'.

Sophie began moving her arms and legs and started coughing. This turned into a cry that gradually became ever more intense and ear piercing. For quite some time she was left to cry, a lonely, desperate cry. I felt her aloneness acutely and I feared that she was hopelessly falling apart. Eliza largely ignored her, playing on the settee with her doll. She did briefly comment that Sophie was crying, walked up to her and stroked her, but quickly moved away again.

Eventually, Michelle came in and without a comment picked Sophie up. The crying stopped and as she offered her a few drops of milk left in the bottle, she greedily sucked, gulping in a lot of air with the milk. As Michelle took the bottle out of her mouth, she started crying again. Michelle put her back in the chair on her own, as she went to prepare more milk. Sophie was again left to cry alone and became ever more frantic. I was afraid that the whole process would be repeated.

From the observation of Sophie, we can see how difficult it can be to let the process take its course, to reflect and to learn but not to 'do anything'. Over time observation enables the observer to tune into and identify with the baby's subjective experience. Ultimately, developing an observational stance can help therapists to imagine and tune into the very earliest relationships and experiences of their (older) child clients and thus make sense of how such happenings impact on their lives in the present. This imagining means reading between the lines of medical files and social work chronologies and background reports. The availability of a robust early history of course makes this task easier, but it is possible to do even when information about the history may be very scant or non-existent, as is often the case with care-experienced children. Holding a lens up to early experiences through current presenting problems may not give a totally accurate picture but may enhance a working hypothesis, making therapists curious about how a children's presenting problems are linked to their earlier experiences.

There are times when the therapeutic situation demands for the therapist to refrain from the urge to intervene actively.

Billy was 8 and in foster care waiting for his 'forever family'. He was extremely active in his sessions, unable to be still, flitting from one activity to the next, leaving little space for thought. Halfway through his session, Billy decided to build a tower with Lego bricks on the floor. With intense concentration he constructed his tower, brick by brick, higher and higher, making it ever more elaborate. He showed great delight in his creation. This was all highly unusual for Billy and the whole process felt precious. It also filled me with anxiety about what would happen next. Inevitably, the last brick was one too many and the whole tower came crashing down.

Billy reacted with extreme despair, threw himself on the floor, rocking in the foetal position. Then, for what seemed like a very long time, Billy sat quietly looking at the heap of bricks, helplessly saying it was all broken and it will never be alright again, everything always went wrong. He was completely deflated and desperate. I sat with him, quietly acknowledging how hard it was when things did not work out. We both knew that this was not just about the tower. There was an overwhelming sense of sadness in the room. As we returned to his foster mother in the waiting room, I told her that Billy would need some extra care today.

(Billy is also referred to later in this chapter)

During this session Billy experienced intense feelings of loss and grief in what Melanie Klein called the depressive position, which may allow us to be in touch with what is not possible and mourn what may never be achieved (Segal 1988). The feelings conveyed were difficult to bear for both child and therapist. The urge for the therapist was to try and take away the pain by suggesting that we could build the tower up again and make everything ok in that moment. Not to do so took enormous effort, not unlike the effort it took to observe baby Sophie without intervening. Reflection in the therapy room allowed the therapist to stay with the child in his grief and for the grief to be acknowledged.

There are other times when therapists literally must think on their feet as the pace dictated by the child is so fast and furious, with many confusing twists and turns. We see this in the example of Jane (see Chapters 4 and 9). Maintaining an observational stance then becomes an extreme challenge and most of the reflecting may need to happen after the session, during the writing up, with colleagues and in supervision.

The importance of early experiences

It is now established knowledge that infant development is experience dependent and that the baby is able to adapt to their emotional environment in the best way for them to ensure their survival (Perry 2006; Zeedyk 2020). For some babies this means being able to develop spontaneously within a loving environment that can eventually support them to explore the outside world, trusting that they will be looked after. For others, whose environment is not in tune with their needs and who experience chronic neglect, abuse and disrupted early relationships, this means developing ways of managing to live with fear and terror. This may involve responding with fight, flight or freeze behaviours. Some children, like baby Sophie, had to adapt to a mother who was often not in tune with her needs. The observer saw her develop into a rather aloof child who did not express distress even when she fell and must have hurt herself. Luckily for Sophie, there were mitigating circumstances, most importantly a supportive relationship with her father, so her development was not considered a major cause for concern. Thus, the baby's emotional, social and physical development is shaped by the nature and quality of their earliest relationship with their care givers. This will impact on the way they are able to find their place in the world and provides a blueprint for future attachment and intimate relationships.

A loving, secure environment does not happen in a vacuum. The parents' own experience of being parented and their own attachment styles impact greatly on how they are able to provide their children with emotional input. Social and economic factors impact on the stress levels in everyday life for parents. Poverty, financial insecurity and social isolation provide the context within which many children grow up. Such external factors, together with more internal, relational factors are important to consider when we as therapists assess children and their families to reach a working formulation.

This recognition about the importance of early infant development and its role in understanding how the child grows is underpinned by ideas developed by psychoanalytic thinkers and practitioners through the ages. It has been strengthened more recently by the emerging evidence of the impact of early experiences on brain development.

Neuroscience

In the last two decades there has been an explosion of knowledge in regard to the early development of the brain, the detrimental impact of neglect and trauma on the developing child and particularly on the neurological development of infants. This knowledge has brought about a coming together of psychological and psychoanalytic theory with neuroscience and child development. Further reading will be required to cover this vast and fascinating area of research and the many theoretical models of intervention it has spawned. For the purposes of this book, we shall focus on a few of the concepts that have most relevance to our practice.

The 'use dependent brain' (Zeedyk 2020) refers to the infant brain developing in response to repeated input and experiences largely within their primary attachment relationships. Those connections that are frequently used are strengthened and fixed into neural pathways and structures, and those not used are pruned away. Prolonged and repeated exposure to circumstances which cause the release of stress hormones without adequate regulation from a caregiver, results in reinforcement of brain pathways alert to danger and high arousal. Thus, stress regulation pathways do not form adequately. The repeated cycle of toxic hormones which flood the brain can result in damage to the developing brain at any stage of childhood, but most particularly in infancy or in utero. This helps us to understand that the children who we see later in their development, may have been impacted by traumatic or neglectful care from their very earliest days, of which they may have no memory.

The Child Trauma Academy is a collection of individuals and organisations working to foster the creation and innovations in practice and policy relating to traumatised and maltreated children. Bruce Perry (2006), one of the co-founders, is an internationally recognised authority on the impact of complex trauma on the developing brain. He has been hugely instrumental in education and influence towards trauma focus worldwide. His Neurosequential Model of Therapeutics (2006) was one of the first intervention models which considered how to assess the areas of the brain where deficits occur, thence intervening with activities in a sequential developmental manner. This could recreate the experiences that would have enabled the development of healthy pathways, had there been an environment without adverse events. While the assessment process within this model is complex,

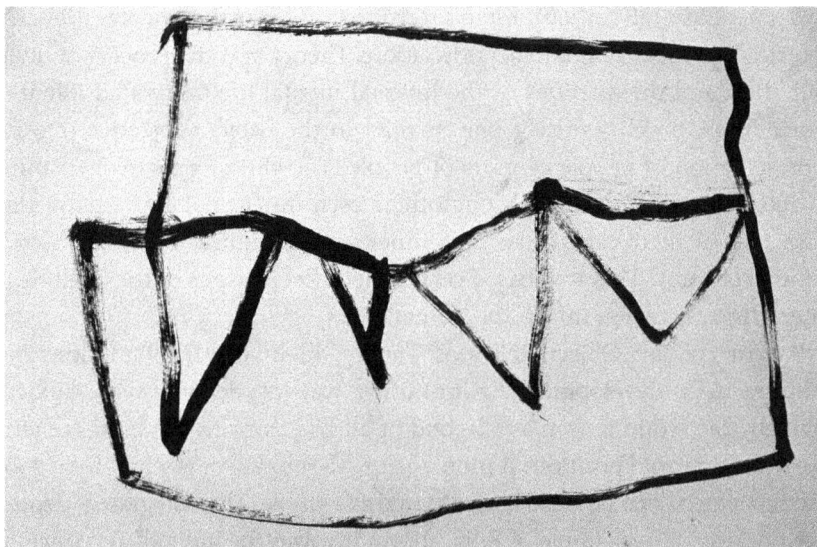

Figure 6.2 'Zig zags' replica artwork based on a drawing by Louis 11 years.

the interventions chime well with our practice of child-led play, where children can safely regress to early play and sensory activities or experiment with sophisticated ideas (Figure 6.2).

The influence of psychoanalytic thinking on play based occupational therapy

It is easy to feel overwhelmed by psychoanalytic writing. Below, we briefly mention psychoanalysts whose ideas have been useful to us.

Sigmund Freud (1856–1939). Known as the 'father of psychoanalysis', Sigmund Freud developed the concept of the unconscious, that is, the idea that human behaviour is as much driven by the unconscious as it is by that which can be seen. His description of the Transference Relationship in therapy continues to be pivotal.

Anna Freud (1895–1982), Sigmund Freud's daughter, was a pioneering child psychoanalyst known for her writings on child development that brought professionals together from many different disciplines. She founded what is now known as The Anna Freud Centre, a major centre for training, research and development.

Melanie Klein (1882–1960). Klein's starting point was that mental life starts at birth. The focus of her Objects Relations Theory was the process of internalisation and the qualities of the internal mental life so created (Shuttleworth 1989, p. 39). Internal objects refer to the baby's subjective internal representation of people or parts of people. The child forms in their mind an internalised landscape, through their own instinctual activity together with that of their caregivers. This inner world acquires a life of its own within the baby. This was based on detailed observations of the minutia of interactions between infant and parent.

As part of her Object Relations Theory, Klein (Segal 1988) described splitting as a developmentally primitive way of dealing with anxiety, whereby the world is seen as all-good or all-bad. For this she used the term 'paranoid-schizoid position'. A more mature development is when both good and bad aspects can be faced and tolerated as a whole. This integrated 'depressive position' (see example of Billy, above) involves the individual mourning the loss of the idealised and accepting that which cannot be changed. It is common to fluctuate between these positions during the course of life.

Donald Winnicott (1896–1971). A decade or so later, the influential psychoanalyst and paediatrician Donald Winnicott (1960a) famously said 'there is no such thing as an infant' meaning that the new-born baby is totally dependent on their caregivers and cannot exist alone. We cannot think about a baby without thinking about the baby *and* someone and about the quality of the care which the baby experiences. The primary care giver, usually the mother, provides an environment of emotional holding (Winnicott 1965) for the baby that, when it is 'good enough' allows the baby to develop a sense of self.

Wilfred Bion (1897–1979). The psychoanalyst Wilfred Bion took Klein's ideas about the psychological development of the infant further and described in detail the containing function of the mother through her 'reverie' – holding the baby in mind through projection, introjection and projective identification (see below). He noted that the mother receiving the baby's projections (e.g., crying) and identifying with the feelings conveyed through this, was the first form of communication between parent and child. Through detailed observations of infants and parents, he developed his theory of thinking. The mother's reverie has parallels with the safety that we are trying to create in the therapeutic relationship. Bion counsels us to approach each session 'without memory or desire' (Symington and

Symington 1996) to allow us as therapists to stay truly in the moment and listen to the child without preconception.

John Bowlby (1907–1990) developed attachment theory. The focus of the child's earliest experiences forms the basis of this. Bowlby's ideas provide a powerful understanding of the importance of consistent, secure infant–parent relationships to promote healthy emotional development. Infants instinctively seek proximity to their caregivers. When care is readily available, children will learn to expect to be safe, which in turn will allow them to explore, and gradually, in adolescence, separate, always knowing that there is a way back. This is in contrast to the children for whom care is more precarious and anxiety provoking.

Mary Ainsworth refined attachment theory into classifications from secure, anxious ambivalent, anxious avoidant and disorganised attachment styles (Ainsworth et al 1978). This forms the basis for many assessment practices. The attachment style of the baby and the toddler has been observed to continue into adulthood, though there are always ways and opportunities for change. The potentially devastating effect of inconsistent, neglectful and abusive early experiences on attachment security and the consequences of this for the child's development is now well understood.

The importance of the above concepts for therapy informed by psychodynamic theories

In individual therapy with children, the therapist tries to understand and tune into the inner world of the child. The dynamics that are played out in the therapy room between a child and their therapist often reflect the child's actual experiences and relationships and how they have learnt to adapt to these. It is often through a reworking of these dynamics in what is known as the transference relationship that healing can take place. Understanding and working with the following theoretical concepts can guide the therapist in this work. These are present in all human communication. We only need to think of how one person's mood can be 'catching' and 'spread'. The intensity of the one-to-one therapeutic relationship allows these processes to be closely observed.

- introjection – taking feelings in/internalising, absorbing feelings and moods

- projection – an unconscious discharging of feelings, ascribing to someone else states of mind in ourselves that we may wish to disown
- projective identification – receiving another person's projections and identifying with them, unconsciously making them our own

These are also the earliest forms of communication between infants and their caregivers (Bion 1962). The baby will project distress or discomfort by crying and the sensitive mother will strive to understand and respond to her baby. In this way a baby can over time, take in a feeling from their 'good enough mother' (Winnicott 1960) who is in tune with their needs. Winnicott coined the term 'the good enough mother' to highlight the idea that ordinary caring parenting meets the baby's needs. Indeed, the perfect parent does not exist. These processes happen naturally without parents needing special psychological insights.

However, as we describe in Chapter 1, the baby who does not have experiences of having their communications understood and responded to, will internalise an absence in the form of 'no mother' (neglect) or a cruel, persecuting mother (abusive). This state of mind for the baby is described by Bion (1962) as 'a nameless dread' and is often linked with debilitating anxiety, leading to fight, flight or freeze responses. We can recognise this internal state of mind in many children who have suffered complex trauma. The task of a therapist is often to receive, hold, think, feel and give back to the child, projections in a modified and manageable form. And just like for the 'good enough mother', these opportunities will come again and again to 'the good enough therapist' during a therapy session or during a course of therapy. In order to respond in this way, the therapist needs to be fully present in the moment.

Transference in the therapeutic relationship refers to feelings and dynamics from past relationships, usually between parent and child, being brought into the therapy room and transferred onto the clinician. This does not refer just to a memory or repetition of earlier relationships, but rather to

> a dynamic and current reliving of feelings and phantasies which in early childhood may never even have been demonstrated or acknowledged.
> (Hoxter 1977, p. 206)

It occurs in the unconscious and is a process based on internalisation, projection and introjection. Melanie Klein emphasised the importance of understanding both positive and negative transference in the therapeutic relationship (Isaacs-Elmhirst 1988). A relationship only becomes real once difficult feelings have been allowed to surface, have been tested and survived. This is demonstrated in the case example of Tanya, earlier discussed in *Occupational Therapy for Child and Adolescent Mental Health* (Ingram 2001, p. 105)

Tanya had been removed from her mother's care following severe sexual abuse and neglect and was living in foster care. The first months of her therapy was characterised by Tanya playing out different aspects of her life in the dolls' house but rarely involving me. Her play seemed detached and repetitive and left me feeling unsure of the value of therapy for Tanya. But when a session had to be cancelled due to illness, Tanya was desperate and furious. Powerful fantasies were unleashed that I had left her so I could be with other children. Overwhelming feelings from the past of rejection and loss, were reawakened and became real. Crucially these feelings now emerged as a feature in the therapy room and could therefore be explored and thought about in the here and now in the transference relationship.

Countertransference covers all feelings that the therapist has in relation to the patient (Heimann 1950, p. 51), rather than simply transference felt by the therapist. Using our observational skills, being fully in the moment allows us to be in tune with what is going on in the room, the spoken word, the felt feelings, the body states of tension or relaxation and how the child may be defending themselves from unbearable feelings. Countertransference is therefore our window to understanding what is going on for our child patients. The therapist needs to work at differentiating which feelings are internal to themselves, originating from their own relationships and experiences and which belong to the patient or to the shared relationship between the therapist and the patient. This shared relationship can be seen as taking place in something akin to the transitional space, described by Winnicott (1971).

Defence mechanisms. As we have seen in Chapter 1, children suffering from complex trauma often develop coping strategies to defend themselves against overwhelming anxiety, for example, denial and rationalisation. Understanding this can help the therapist tune into children's emotional states.

Some children use apparently pointless activity, something akin to playing, to manage their anxiety by cutting themselves off from connection with the world. This forms an internal wall and children who have experienced complex trauma may need this as protection from their external world and their internal demons. Graham Music (2022) advocates respecting such walls.

> New understandings of trauma explain why it can be vital to tiptoe slowly up to pain, or even sidestep, pain. First of all, we need to build safety-based feeling states that help turn down danger signals. Traumatised people need safety first. Putting them in touch with their trauma too quickly can be like prodding an open wound with a sharp instrument, triggering re-traumatisation and redoubling defences such as dissociative states and flashbacks.
>
> (Music, p. 30)

Returning to Billy in this chapter, building his Lego tower, had many sessions which were characterised by a rather manic flitting from activity to activity without being able to settle to anything. There was a sense of hopelessness and futility about the sessions that in turn left the therapist, in the countertransference, feeling rather useless, wondering about the merits of continuing therapy. This can be understood as Billy unconsciously but successfully making sure that nothing of meaning was touched upon in the sessions, holding at bay unbearable anxiety about his future. His defences were strong. The hopelessness was instead transferred onto the therapist who felt this acutely, through projective identification. It was not until the tower he built came crashing down that the defensive wall also disintegrated, and he was able to allow himself to be vulnerable. The therapist decided to stay within the theme of his tower rather than directly making a link with his external situation. Their hunch was that naming his anxiety about his future would likely have propelled him back into his defensiveness, whereas staying with his despair in the moment was more helpful.

Systemic understanding

It is important to recognise the contribution of systemic ideas to individual therapeutic work with children. Systemic theory is based on the belief that problems and difficulties can be viewed in an interpersonal way whereby experience is fundamentally relational rather than individual. This means a shift from linear to circular causation of understanding presenting difficulties (Vetere and Dallos 2003). As we have seen, the lives of children with complex trauma are often characterised by chaotic family circumstances and multiple placements. Involvement of a large system of professional networks is commonplace. It is crucial that such systems can work together to reach a common language so that we can find jointly understood formulations, whereby therapy can be seen as one piece of a jigsaw that makes up the support for the child.

Being clear about the parameters around the sessions in terms of time, space, regularity, length of therapy, who brings the child and how people in the child's life can be supportive of the therapy without being intrusive, is part of the important preparation that may take considerable time and effort. This process itself can be helpful when assessing whether the timing and conditions for therapy for a particular child are right, or, put another way, whether there is what Monica Lanyado, child psychotherapist (1991) calls, sufficient external therapeutic space that can be maintained through the course of therapy and not just at the start. Louise Emanuel (2002) explored how the trauma and disturbance associated with severe neglect and abuse in children impacts on the systems of which they are a part, rendering professionals and organisations unable to think clearly. This process can be seen as a re-enactment of the original neglect and is akin to the 'freeze reaction' that can be seen in disorganised attachment. Similarly, Boswell and Cudmore (2017) talk about collective blindness in the system when the needs of the individual child can be lost, and decisions become resource-led instead of child-led.

Therapists therefore need to be mindful of their own agency, their responsibilities and boundaries, so that they can influence decision-making in the system in professional and ethical ways when needed. This can at times take considerable courage and effort. Even if there aren't the resources it is important to state and hold on to the child's needs. In the face of such dynamics, therapists need supported within their own organisations to hold the position of the child's experience.

The MOVI model of occupational therapy – similarities and differences with PBOT

This section begins with a description of MOVI, as a useful framework. Central to MOVI is the therapeutic relationship as connected by the activity or the 'doing'. There are parallels between PBOT, as we define it, and MOVI, with its emphasis on the dynamic interaction between the patient, the therapist and the 'doing', or as we see it, the 'playing'. This threesome can be imagined as a triangle.

The use of activity is central to all contemporary occupational therapy models. MOVI differs by placing a strong emphasis on the relationship and being significantly influenced by psychoanalytic theory. This of course chimes well with PBOT where play is the activity, and the therapist utilises an understanding of unconscious communication and processes.

MOVI was developed by Italian occupational therapists Julie Piergrossi and Carolina Gibertoni de Sena and described in their book *Psychanalytic Thinking in Occupational Therapy* (Nicholls et al. 2013). It is a relational model for practice across the age range, children to adults, which emphasises the unconscious process taking place within the relationship between client and therapist during an activity or 'doing' as they refer. The 'doing' allows access to the client's thoughts, feelings and unconscious processes, making them available to be considered, explored and perhaps interpreted.

In MOVI the activities of doing can be creative, or more practical, such as cooking. Choosing the activity is part of the interactive therapeutic process. The model considers that the act of doing can be transformational within the containment of the therapist's reflective presence.

Both MOVI and PBOT underline the importance of the therapeutic setting where transformation can occur in many areas: emotions, materials, sensory experiences and thoughts.

The following example demonstrates the 'Materials and Transformation' element of MOVI practice (Nicholls et al. 2013, p. 120)

Jake aged 8, was living in foster care. The carer had informed me prior to his session that Jake had met with his older brother that week, who he had not seen for several weeks since the children were received into care. I told Jake that I knew about him meeting his brother and wondered how it had been for him. 'Oh ok' he replied in a cheerful tone that didn't give anything away and didn't invite further enquiry. He wanted to play with the clay again and quietly set to work making a small pot. I could do the same.

The pots were to have lids, and it was important that they fitted over the top so that nothing fell out. Once there were several pots that he was happy with, he started to make little balls of clay that he placed inside. The number of balls in each pot was important as he counted and recounted. He began to balance each pot on top of the other, becoming concerned that balancing required the pots to be squished down into each other and that the lids were buckling and pots losing shape. He expressed a worry that the balls inside were getting squashed. As the tower of pots was teetering, losing shape and his anxiety escalating, he suddenly jumped out of his seat and pushed the whole construction down.

He pounded the misshapen pots with his fist. After a moment or two he stopped and peeled off the remains of a lid. Underneath he picked out the clay that had made up two of the balls. Carefully, from the remains, he made two little people, one noticeably bigger than the other.

The therapist understood that Jake would find it difficult to express his very complicated feelings about his older brother and his birth family, that were likely reignited by the recent reunion. The themes of safety, care, containment, anxiety, anger, destruction and attachment, seemed all to be present in his play and within the transference. Transformation of these themes into the clay, and within the context of the therapeutic relationship, would allow these difficult feelings to be thought about and processed.

We have found it most encouraging to finally have an occupational therapy model with which we can identify, and which highlights the emotions in the relationship as central. While there are significant similarities between MOVI and PBOT, there are also fundamental differences in how we practice. Piergrossi and Gibertoni de Sena work in private practice with a different clientele and without the resource pressures of the NHS in the UK. The needs of the vulnerable children we work with require a whole system approach which is not yet developed for MOVI based work.

There is a developing body of literature on MOVI extending out of Milan through to Brunel University. The existing community of practitioners see Edinburgh CAMHS and those practicing PBOT as a centre of 'like mindedness'.

Person-centred therapy and PBOT

Therapists over the years have been inspired by the ground-breaking work of Virginia Axline, an early play therapist who adapted Carl Rodgers' person centred technique of counselling to work with children through non-directive play. In her short book, *Dibs in Search of Self* (1964), Axline relates how play therapy can have a profound impact on one child's emotional and intellectual development. She devised eight basic principles of non-directive play therapy that guided her work (Axline 1989). Whereas these principles may seem dated in today's pressurised clinical environments with clearly defined time constraints and requirements for outcome measures, we believe that they have their place as a practice guide for forming therapeutic relationships with children. More recent developments in understanding of neuropsychology and complex trauma have led us to understand that non-directive therapy alone is not sufficient to help children process and recover from trauma. Rather, therapy needs to be trauma-focused even though it is child-led. It is helpful for the child to know that the therapist is informed of and can hold in mind what has happened to them and of some of their presenting difficulties. Child-led means that the therapist is in tune with and respectful of how the child chooses to communicate in the session, both when the content is initiated wholly by the child and when the therapist has initiated parts of the session to include structured activities, such as family drawings (see Chapter 5). The therapy takes place against the backdrop of the child's experiences and external environment in the here and now. Axline's principles powerfully compliment a sound understanding of trauma-informed therapy and of psychodynamic and systemic ideas and help the therapist develop unconditional positive regard for their child clients. They lend themselves to be modified when working with a specific focus on complex trauma.

Axline's eight principles of play therapy:

1. The therapist must develop a warm friendly relationship with the child, in which good rapport is established as soon as possible.
2. The therapist accepts the child exactly as he is.
3. The therapist establishes a feeling of permissiveness in the relationship so that the child feels free to express his feelings completely.
4. The therapist is alert to recognise the feelings the child is expressing and reflects those feelings back in such a manner that the child gains insight into his behaviour.
5. The therapist maintains a deep respect for the child's ability to solve his own problems if given an opportunity to do so. It is the responsibility of the child to make choices and to institute change.

6. The therapist does not attempt to direct the child's actions or conversations in any manner. The child leads the way; the therapist follows.
7. The therapist does not attempt to hurry the therapy along. It is a gradual process and is recognised as such by the therapist.
8. The therapist establishes only those limitations that are necessary to anchor the therapy to the world of reality and to make the child aware of his responsibility in the relationship.

Reference list

Ainsworth, M.D.S., Blehar, M.C., Waters, E., Wall, S. (1978). *Patterns of Attachment: A Psychological Study of the Strange Situation*. Earlbaum.

Axline, V.M. (1964). *Dibs in Search of Self*. Pelican.

Axline, V.M. (1989). *Play Therapy*, 2nd ed. Churchill Livingstone.

Bick, E. (1964). Notes on infant observation in psychoanalytic training. *International Journal of Psychoanalysis*, 45, 558–566.

Bion, W. (1962). A theory of thinking. *International Journal of Psychoanalysis*, 43, 306–310.

Boswell, S., Cudmore, L. (2017). Understanding the 'blind spot' when children move from foster care into adoption. *Journal of Child Psychotherapy*, 43 (2), 243–257.

Emanuel, L. (2002). Deprivation 2 3. *Journal of Child Psychotherapy*, 28 (2), 163–179.

Heimann, P. (1950). On counter-transference. *International Journal of Psychoanalysis*, 31, 81–84.

Hoxter, S. (1977). Play and communication. In Boston, M., Daws, D. eds. *The Child Psychotherapist and Problems of Young People*. Wildwood House, p. 206.

Ingram, G. (2001). Psychodynamic theories. In Lougher, L. ed. *Occupational Therapy for Child and Adolescent Mental Health*. Churchill Livingstone, p. 105.

Isaacs-Elmhirst, S. (1988). The Kleinian setting for child analysis. *International Review of Psychoanalysis*, 15, 5–12.

Lanyado, M. (1991). On creating a psychotherapeutic space. *Journal of Social Work Practice*, 5 (1), 31–40.

Music, G. (2022). *Respark: Igniting Spark and Joy after Trauma and Depression*. Mind-Nurturing Books.

Nicholls, L., Piergrossi, J.C., Gibertoni, C.deS., Daniel, M., eds. (2013). *Psychoanalytic Thinking in Occupational Therapy*. Wiley-Blackwell, pp. 105–127.

Perry, B.D. (2006). The neurosequential model of therapeutics: Applying principles of neuroscience to clinical work with traumatised and maltreated children. In Webb, N.B. ed. *Working with Traumatized Youth in Child Welfare*. The Guildford Press, pp. 27–52.

Segal, H. (1988). *Introduction to the Work of Melanie Klein*. Karnac.

Shuttleworth, J. (1989). Psychoanalytic theory and infant development. In Miller L. et al. eds. *Closely Observed Infants*. Duckworth, pp. 22–51.

Symington, J., Symington, N. (1996). *The Clinical Thinking of Wilfred Bion*. Routledge, pp. 166–174.

Vetere, A., Dallos, R. (2003). *Working Systemically with Families: Formulation, Intervention and Evaluation*. Karnac.

Winnicott, D.W. (1960). The theory of the parent-infant relationship. *International Journal of Psychoanalysis*, 41, 585–595.

Winnicott, D.W. (1965). *The Family and Individual Development*. Tavistock.

Winnicott, D.W. (1971). *Playing and Reality*. Routledge.

Zeedyk, S. (2020). *Sabre Tooth Tigers and Teddy Bears: The Connected Baby Guide to Attachment*. Connected Baby Ltd.

7

THE THERAPEUTIC PROCESS

At the beginning of the therapeutic process, the main aim is to develop a trusting relationship between the therapist and the child. This entails orienting the child and their parent to what they can expect, along the lines described previously. How this is done will vary depending on the child's developmental age. The child will need to experience how it feels *to be with* the therapist. It may take a few sessions before they are able to make sense of the boundaries of the sessions and issues to do with confidentiality. Hopefully a containing relationship can be formed which can withstand challenges, disappointments and strong emotions linked with both positive and negative transference which will surely enter the room in future sessions.

The middle phase is when the real work takes place. During this time, it can be difficult to know what is going on both in the therapeutic relationship and in the child's play, which may be confusing. Progress may be hard to gauge. Sessions may be challenging, and the therapist may struggle to know how to proceed. Managing practical difficulties like maintaining

DOI: 10.4324/9781003642862-8

safety can be complex. Sessions may even seem meaningless and boring, without much happening. They may seem 'artificially nice', giving rise to questions about what is being avoided. Staying with not knowing becomes important (Lanyado and Horne 1999, p. 66). This middle phase is also when transformative things can happen. Faith in the power of the therapeutic process must be maintained by the therapist. Themes may begin to emerge.

The therapist watched with bated breath when a child who had spent many sessions angrily breaking up Playmobil vehicles into tiny pieces, suddenly began creating a new 'ambulance' out of fire engine wheels, police car roof etc. Out of pieces of destruction this child created a new 'whole', something integrated and different.

Knowing when a child with complex trauma is ready to stop therapy can be difficult. Afterwards many children will need different ongoing support. Lanyado and Horne (1999) suggest that there comes a stage in the therapeutic relationship when it must be left behind, as its 'purpose has been served' (p. 71). They point to the parallel between the letting go in ordinary parenting because it is developmentally timely to do so, and the ending of therapy. Quite often the child communicates in some way that they are ready to stop, as with a boy who took his toys out of his box and lined them up on the windowsill 'ready for other children to play with'.

Ending therapy must be thought about from the start. Giving sufficient time for the ending is important so that strong feelings about the impending separation can be contained in the therapy room. Whilst we have formulated general aims of therapy, it is not possible to predict exactly what the outcome will be (Lanyado 1999). There is a risk in busy departments that therapists feel a need to bring therapy to a close prematurely after some initial improvement. Children with complex trauma have usually been subject to losses which have been sudden and distressing. Ending therapy in a planned and thoughtful way can give the child an opportunity to experience a transition where feelings of rejection and abandonment can be worked through. Mourning the loss of therapy can help the child internalise the goodness of the therapeutic relationship.

Children manage the ending period differently. Making the ending tangible by keeping a counting down diary can help. Some children quite systematically go through what they have played with during their time in therapy. One child who had moved placements several times during therapy, wanted to be reminded about what they had played with when they lived in different places. Some children ask to have an ending 'party', or to be able to take a token toy with them from the therapy room. This needs to be done sensitively to maintain the significance of the ending.

Views amongst therapists vary about how to deal with artwork and other creations which the child has produced. Some children are told that they can take their paintings home. Other therapists view what has been produced in therapy as belonging to the therapeutic relationship and therefore, risks losing its meaning by being taken home. Will it be kept safe or will it end up under the bed, chewed by the dog or scribbled on by little sister? Our view is that the expectations about what happens to such material should be clear at the onset so as not to overshadow the ending. The focus needs to remain on the separation and how the child can take in what the relationship has brought.

Sudden and unprepared endings bring a big challenge. This is when therapists need to consider what mitigating measures can be put in place, such as letters, indirect contact through carers or professionals still involved, or maybe even some online meetings.

Two cases

The following case descriptions of longer-term play based occupational therapy (PBOT) with Rory and Kenneth offer an opportunity to think about the beginning, middle and end of the therapeutic process. Each case starts with information about the child's background and reason for referral. Descriptions of some aspects of the therapy sessions, written in the first person, follow. Finally, there are reflections and discussion of the impact of therapy.

RORY

Rory aged 7, was removed from his mother at birth, and after three foster placements was adopted aged 3. He was referred to Child and Adolescent Mental Health Services (CAMHS) due to concerns about dysregulated, aggressive behaviour towards his parents and teachers. He could not sleep on his own. He needed 1:1 support for most of the school day. His peer relationships were difficult, often resulting in fights. Rory was developmentally young for his age. His is an example of a child using PBOT to work through developmental stages of play and relating. In the 18 months of therapy, he developed from a boy with little independence from his parents to a much more self-assured boy who could hold his own both at home and at school.

BEGINNING

During the assessment phase, Rory mostly played alone with no representational play or role play, sometimes leaving me feeling completely superfluous. Play gradually developed into more reciprocal communication, with us rolling the ball backwards and forwards, initially in a quiet rhythmic way. Rory would then increase the intensity and force of the ball game. His play often became physically aggressive either towards the puppets or me and he needed occasional reminding of our rules such as 'you can't hurt the room, yourself or me'. When his session ended each week, he often needed reassurance that he would return to the same room the following week. Below is his response to being reminded of a week's break and the forthcoming review meeting with parents to discuss continuation of therapy (Figure 7.1):

Rory picked up the puppet turtle and made a whining noise. I wondered if it was worried, and Rory nodded. I reminded him we had a few minutes left. He started shaking the turtle's head and throwing it to the ground with great force and then against the wall. His aggression took me by surprise, perhaps he was surprised to be told of his remaining time. He picked up the puppet dragon and swung it round, bashed it against the wall and used it as a whip which narrowly missed me. His aggression towards the puppets was disturbing to watch. I felt sad and powerless and commented that 'it feels really sad and frustrating' and wondered aloud if it was difficult to finish. I reminded him that he and I and his parents would have a think about what should happen next and whether he needed to see me for a bit longer. He instructed me, 'ask the turtle more or less'. I asked the turtle whilst looking at Rory, clarifying 'more sessions?' Both turtle and Rory affirmed with a nod. I thanked them for letting me know.

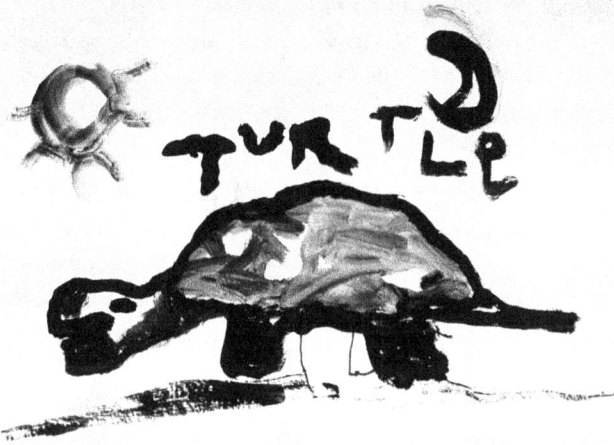

Figure 7.1 'The turtle' replica artwork based on a painting by Rory 7 years.

My reflection

Rory's level of aggression towards the puppets and me was unexpected and might have reflected his anxiety about the uncertainty about continuing therapy. His behaviour overall was a challenge for me to manage (Figure 7.1). I worried about both his and my safety. It was hard to keep a thinking space in my mind and not immediately to rush to remind him that we need to stay safe. Sometimes I acknowledged that he was 'giving me a hard time'. Through progression of therapy, I tried to avoid joining in this 'dance' of attack and rejection.

MIDDLE

During the middle phase of the therapy Rory tended to move around a lot, particularly at the beginning and end of sessions. His vigorous activity included extremely physical ball play but also sensory play, mixing play dough, sometimes adding to it sand and paper, as shown by the two following excerpts

Rory threw the ball back to me using his fists, head, whole body, sometimes rolling on it and landing on the floor. He complained of hurting himself.

I acknowledged that he wanted me to notice he was hurt. This seemed to slow him down. Whenever I moved towards him, he moved away. Perhaps he found me intrusive or the idea of close physical contact between us might have felt overwhelming.

Rory had been flitting from one activity to another in this session. He took his multi-coloured ball of play dough from his box and started to break it into many pieces. This game developed a momentum. He hid the pieces all over the playroom and asked me to help him find them. We searched high and low almost like a game of peek-a-boo, reflecting on their different shapes, sizes and colours. When they were all gathered up and squashed together Rory stood back and admired the shape. He referred to it as a colourful jewel. We looked at it together. This was a moment of real connection. We spoke of its transformation from little lumps to a jewel.

My reflection

This process seemed reminiscent of Bion's (1962) container/contained relationship where the scattered and seemingly senseless bits and pieces are received and thought about by the therapist and thence transformed into something more coherent and with meaning. This felt like an expression of different parts of Rory which were being gathered up and put together in a different way. Interestingly, this theme continued throughout his therapy.

I wondered about his need for constant movement and his poor impulse control in the beginning. Was it a defence against thinking about painful early experiences? His dysregulation had gradually lessened until he could stay with a play theme for much longer and develop it. Now that he was less active, I was able to notice what was happening. He was slowly beginning to involve me more. He was more interested in relating to me, instructing me to take part in role play, albeit often on an opposing team which placed me under attack.

When working with children who have had minimal early containment, Copley and Forryan (1997) explain that: 'the worker must also expect to be attacked as the transference representation of an earlier object for not fulfilling this function' (p. 250). Paradoxically, Rory was keen to come to therapy, referring to it as 'paradise', yet he was critical and attacking towards me. However, it seemed that if I could pay close attention to his play and receive his projections, Rory could then take in and make use of this containing experience. The excerpt below shows in a concrete way how this was beginning to happen

Rory made pizza with his play dough and offered me a piece. He lay down on the beanbag and asked me to sit next to him. We both enjoyed 'eating' the pizza and feeding each other. It was as if we were taking in a little piece of each other.

Rory had begun to share his internal world. The hope was that he could then begin to risk forming new attachments where feelings can be safely expressed. Kenrick et al. (2019) describe this process:

> Previous negative attachment models and their associated feelings can then be expressed in a context in which they are acknowledged in words, not by enactment.
>
> (p. 105)

ENDING

Preparing for the ending, I was aware that both Rory and his parents needed to feel ready. Rory's parents were anxious about letting go and risking a regression in his behaviour. Rory was doing well in his external world. He was no longer needing extra support within school. He was managing transitions well and was sleeping in his own bed. He was getting on much better with his peers and could even take part in extracurricular sport activities. In spite of this I acknowledged with parents that it would be hard for him to stop therapy and that setbacks were likely. Nevertheless, it would be important for him to feel able to manage without a therapist.

Rory's weekly sessions were spaced out to be fortnightly for a while. This facilitated his ability to slowly let go. During our last weeks, his attacking behaviours towards me became less extreme. Before a session ended, he would often seek a solution to the destructive play, or he would invite me to 'join his team'. Rory and his parents were given three 'family tokens' which they could use during the following 12 months. This way they would have the opportunity to touch base with me albeit in a space different from the playroom and with Rory and parents together. His parents told me they felt it had been helpful for Rory to experience the emotional risk of trusting an adult who was different from them. They did not choose to use the family tokens.

KENNETH

Kenneth aged 13, was referred with harmful sexual behaviour which included touching his private parts in public, thrusting his hips at his carer and teachers, and use of sexualised language towards other children. Since the death of his mother from cancer three years ago, his older sister Hailey (25 years) decided to take on the care of her brother. At home Kenneth had witnessed domestic violence over some years perpetrated by his father towards his mother. The couple separated when Kenneth was eight years old and contact with his father ceased abruptly. Two years later apparently in response to sex education at school he disclosed sexual abuse by his father and other males, which more recently he had denied. Hailey's own childhood and young adulthood had been characterised by years of violence and abuse. Initially Kenneth also witnessed some domestic violence towards Hailey by her previous partners. However, motivated by her wish to turn her life around and to care for her younger brother, soon after their mother's death she ceased all contact with her previous abusive partners.

Kenneth was socially and emotionally immature and struggled to learn at school. He showed impulsive, disruptive and aggressive behaviour. Despite attending a special educational provision and despite intensive input and monitoring by Social Work in consultation with our team, change was proving hard to achieve. Sex education and work on body boundaries were embarked on at school. Hailey was supported to explain and adhere to boundaries at home. She agreed that Kenneth would attend CAMHS for six weeks of play based sessions for assessment. Transport to our department was provided by Social Work. Following that period Kenneth's Social Worker would be involved in feedback and discussion about the next step.

Meetings with CAMHS, social work and educational professionals were frequent throughout our contact. Child Protection reviews were regular. As is often the case it is difficult to know what type of input is most helpful at what moment. Hailey was building up a trusting relationship with the social worker which was essential to support any progress for her and for Kenneth. She found it difficult to reflect on her own childhood, just referring to that time as 'dreadful'. Three family members were currently in prison. As Kenneth began to meet with me, Hailey was supported to engage in therapy with a domestic abuse agency.

BEGINNING

Initial individual session

During a previous meeting with Hailey and again on the phone I had 'rehearsed' with her, what she might tell Kenneth about his first appointment with me. Despite this, it was apparent that she had not managed to tell him anything more than the appointment time. He only knew that our department was part of the hospital.

When I went to collect him, I greeted Kenneth, a tall boy with pale skin and acne. I tried to clarify that this was not a hospital department where we would x-ray him, do injections or put on plasters. I said that this was a place where he and I can play or paint and think together. He might find that he thinks about good times or that he thinks about times which have been difficult. I explained that he and I would go upstairs together and after about 45 minutes I would bring him back to his sister who would be waiting to take him home.

As Kenneth and I were about to leave the corridor, Hailey started telling the story of their arrival at the department. She said they were brought by the social worker who left them 'miles away' in an unfamiliar area. She said she had difficulty breathing and that no one could help her. Her anxiety gave little space for Kenneth. Despite getting lost, Kenneth and Hailey had arrived 30 minutes early, and not wishing to go into the waiting room, sat in the cold corridor. I suggested Hailey might like to keep warm in the waiting room while Kenneth came with me. She didn't move. It appeared that Hailey searched out situations where she could feel unnoticed or even an outcast.

Both Hailey and Kenneth seemed uncertain of what was expected of them. As if to escape such discomfort Kenneth quickly stood up and left his sister. He accompanied me, jumping up three stairs at a time. Once in the playroom he seized two small balls and with a voice of authority began teaching me how to juggle. It seemed that he felt a need to take control. I told him how hard I found this game. Feeling uncomfortable I said, 'I can't seem to learn how to juggle. I'm feeling really stupid. You are showing me how it feels not to manage.'

My reflection

I tried to contain Hailey's anxiety in order for Kenneth to more easily separate from her. I felt vividly her fragility and isolation. It was several weeks later that she was able to explain on the phone that she was terrified that she would lose Kenneth, and he would be taken away into foster care.

In the playroom I knew I would fail in the juggling lesson. In the countertransference I felt worried and helpless, and even disabled in my complete inability to even start. This was interesting in the light of a recent request from school to assess Kenneth for intellectual disability.

MIDDLE

Following the initial assessment and review, PBOT sessions continued for 12 months. Occasionally, Kenneth embarked on inappropriate activity such as removing his shirt or thrusting his groin at me. In response I let Kenneth know I could see what he was doing and gave words to describe it. I explained and repeated rules such as 'we keep our clothes on in this room' and 'it's against the rules to push your hips towards me'. At times I wondered with him, not expecting an answer, what had happened to him to make him behave in this way.

Kenneth seemed keen to come to each of his weekly sessions. After ten sessions, I explained to him that I would be away for two weeks and so he will miss two appointments.

Kenneth looked downcast but said nothing. I commented on him perhaps feeling fed up. He nodded. We were both quiet. After a while I said that I was wondering if he thinks he won't come back here. He didn't respond. I stressed to him that after the break we would have more sessions. 'Oh good' Kenneth said, 'I like coming here.'

Kenneth then found a toy dinosaur which he held on my shoulder, making loud growling sounds into my ear. I felt some alarm and said that the dinosaur was scary. Kenneth responded by moving the dinosaur, so its head touched my cheek. I immediately felt relieved and moved by this noisy boy's ability to be so gentle. It was quiet in the room, and I said, 'the dinosaur is now so gentle. He was growly at first then he changed.' I couldn't quite trust this to continue and wondered where this might lead. I voiced this to Kenneth, 'I can't trust the dinosaur because I know what he can be like.'

Apparently out of the blue, Kenneth said, 'I told my Dad to go away and leave Mum and me alone. So, Dad went.' He became unusually still and reminded me of a much younger boy. I wondered aloud about him feeling sad and perhaps having tried to look after his Mum. I wondered how he felt now about his Dad leaving. Did he feel he had done the right thing? He replied, 'we don't talk about what happens in the family.' Although this sounded like a phrase he might have heard elsewhere, he was also telling me that there were family secrets. It was an effective way for him to emotionally close down. It left no space for me to mention the subsequent death of his mother and how that might have affected him.

He immediately stopped the dinosaur game and returned to his more usual noisy, active and controlling play in the sand tray. He hurtled the cars around a track, with the 'winning' cars jumping right out of the sand, some almost hitting me. Kenneth had regained his power. That day he resisted leaving the therapy room, shouting that he had more time and that the clock was wrong and, 'you are wrong!' I wondered if I had missed a vital moment to give him space to articulate feelings about the loss of his mother.

My reflection

I found myself wondering how I could ever help Kenneth to move on from all his accumulation of trauma. How could we ever establish an even relationship between us as fellow humans? Sessions felt like a battle for control, him to control me and me to control him in order to keep us both safe. To acknowledge his vulnerability seemed cruel and for me to speak of my vulnerability was not appropriate.

Kenneth chose activities similar to those of a much younger child, such as pushing cars around the sand tray. Maybe such developmentally young activities felt comfortable for him. There was little imaginative play. His stories had a sense of paucity and emptiness about them. How could he begin to process his trauma into a narrative if there were secrets that could not be allowed out into the open?

The mixed tenderness and aggression shown by the dinosaur might have indicated a way forward. At some time, he must have experienced such confusingly mixed emotions. Beyond the sexual abuse which he had alleged, I wondered at the likelihood of his witnessing or being caught up in adult sexual behaviour in the past or even currently. The question of how he could grow up to be a mature, balanced, safe male was ever present.

In Kenneth's 29th session he told me to act being a young girl Stella, who returns home from school to tell her big brother what had happened to her. Kenneth took the role of the big brother. The story was that I (Stella) had been sexually assaulted 'in a creepy way'. He described what action he took, 'I ran out of the house and battered the guy and ditched him.' This was acted out using imaginative play with extreme violence though amazingly he managed not to hurt either himself or me.

He told me (Stella) that I was not to tell our Mum what had happened.

I (Stella) asked, 'why not?'

'Because I want to live alone in a big house because Mum loves you Stella, more than me.' He rapidly continued to tell the story. 'The brother then went away to fight a war. When he returned, he came to rescue Mum and Stella.'

I asked, 'Why is he rescuing us?'

He replied, 'Dad has killed 35 children and he's on his way to kill you both.'

This disjointed story shows several powerful themes which puzzled me and were difficult to disentangle. Omnipotence and violence were always present. Confusion about his protective role for the family seemed like a web holding Kenneth in a position which was hard to change.

By the time of this story of Stella, Kenneth had been coming to PBOT for ten months.

I found that the moments of connection with Kenneth were few. We had reached a very low point and my hope for change was diminishing. Recognising this in supervision was a shock to me. I resolved to really look for tiny changes in the room, what Kenneth says and does and how he says it, even amidst his excessive activity.

Following a phone call with the social worker to share some of these feelings, the network around Kenneth and I seemed to come alive, as if they heard my despair. The social worker told me that Hailey was completely engaged in her own therapy. Kenneth's teachers at school spontaneously phoned to tell me about Kenneth's improved behaviour and his increased ability to focus on his work, including the adapted syllabus on sex and relationships. His sexualised behaviour towards other children was reducing. This 'holding' process in the complex support system around Kenneth encouraged in me realistic optimism about Kenneth's potential to progress. I could see that he had invested in the relationship with me and me with him. Lanyado and Horne (1999) write of the subtlety of this dilemma

> It can be surprising to find that there are times when the understanding remains with the therapist and is never put into words and yet there is significant change in the child's relationships and level of disturbance.
>
> (p. 66)

The professional team around Kenneth and his sister agreed to an assessment of Kenneth for attention-deficit/hyperactivity disorder and intellectual disability. This resulted in a diagnosis of both conditions and a trial of medication. He understood this as a way 'to help him change his brain'. Liaison between services, our team and school continued (Figure 7.2).

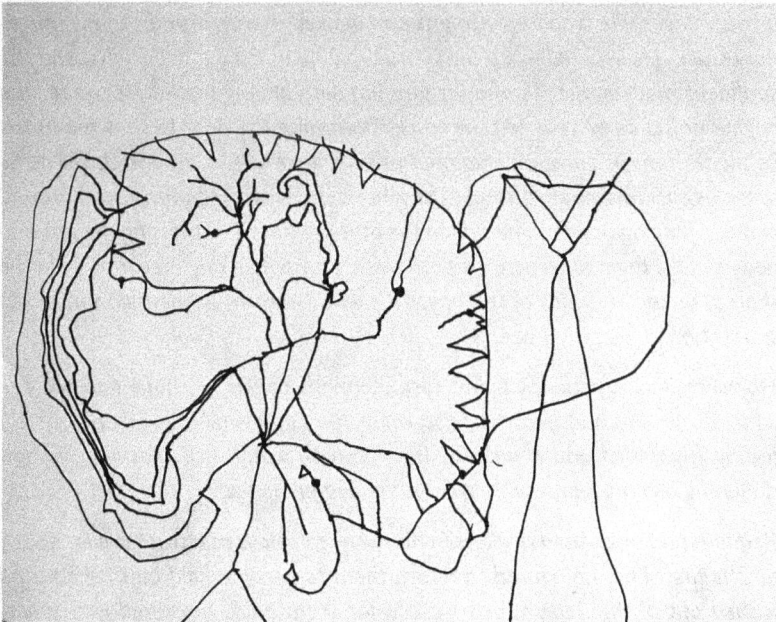

Figure 7.2 'My brain' replica artwork based on a painting by Kenneth 13 years.

ENDING

Right from the first meetings with Kenneth, as with all children, I indicated that these sessions will eventually end. When he had attended for nine months, and I reminded him of this, he told me that he wanted ten more sessions before we say goodbye. So, there was a countdown each week. As finishing time came closer, he stated he wanted 300 more sessions. At this time, he painted the image he named 'My Growing Heart', depicted on the front cover of this book. The ending of sessions proved challenging and seemed to pull us apart. He seemed emotionally insatiable. In order to help him manage his pain with some dignity, I told him how many minutes were left of each session; ten minutes left, five, two, one and then finish. Kenneth, who of course had experienced several unexpected losses of close relationships, needed particular help to contemplate ending. He was aware that the ending of each session was a rehearsal for the end of our contact.

In his penultimate appointment Kenneth borrowed my keys for his play as a truck driver. He stood up straight and walked, hands on hips to his imaginary truck. He seemed like a large man, giving himself a deep voice and the confident movements of someone familiar with driving trucks. He made loud engine noises as he reversed the truck, slamming the door to shut me in the cab with him. In our joint imaginations we were tossed up and down as he drove us over imaginary bumps. The wheels shrieked as the truck sped around corners, flinging us from one side to the other. We were witnessing the ups and downs of life together. There we both were, bumping along precariously in the shared, unknown space of therapy. This was surely an authentic moment of connection.

However, this experience didn't last. Kenneth began to shout and tell me what to do. He had become once more the aggressor. I was at his mercy, feeling frightened and powerless. But Kenneth would hear nothing of that, drowning out my words with ever louder engine noises.

Kenneth had often used my keys in his many roleplays as a truck driver. Today for the first time, he refused to return them to me. He held on to them and rushed out of the door. When I asked for them back, he stared into space, refusing to engage with me. He rushed downstairs, out of the building and across the road.

Hailey, noticing us had joined us by the busy road and she called to him to return my keys. After refusing and arguing he suddenly threw them to me, as he darted into the traffic. She called him and he immediately returned to the pavement and fell into a hug with her. Previously when Kenneth was upset, she would try to jolly him out of his misery. In complete contrast today she asked him what was bothering him, suggesting he might be angry as his time coming here was ending next week. I was astonished by her ability to understand and be in touch with his feelings when previously she had found this so difficult. I suggested he might be sad as well as angry. He turned to me and for the first time ever he hugged me. He was tearful and buried his head in my shoulder. I told him I too was sad. As we went inside to collect his jacket, he explained that he had taken my keys so as to be able to let himself in to our building in order to see me once his appointments had ended.

During Kenneth's final session, his role play lacked its previous noise and vigour, leaving me wishing I had more ideas on how to manage. I commented how hard it is to know what to do now, when for months we've worked so hard together. Kenneth agreed, saying that we had already said goodbye. How right he was. He then laughed at his own wish to keep my keys. I was able to tell him I would remember him. He did not meet my eyes. Finally, he darted out of the room and down the stairs to his sister. She allowed me to gently touch her arm as we said goodbye.

My reflection

During his penultimate session I felt stupid to have let Kenneth use my keys and humiliated at my inability to keep him safe. The road was dangerous. I use the word 'stupid' deliberately to reflect how I felt in the countertransference. It fits with Kenneth's constant struggle to think about the world and relationships. Stupidity and humiliation were both feelings familiar to Kenneth but to bring those words into our sessions had been difficult.

Thinking about the months of work with Kenneth, his need to control every aspect of each session was exhausting: the time, the activity, the rules of his games. His role plays usually required him to be omnipotent, the boss, whilst he placed me in role of underling or the 'woman'. I found it was difficult not to add to his distress by putting into words my understanding of his 'real world'. Once, for example, I referred to his absconding from school and his sister's worry for his safety. He stared at me, rigid and silent. Even my efforts to tiptoe up to the pain, as Graham Music (2022, p. 30) so gently writes, felt clunky and cruel.

Kenneth's efforts to negotiate ongoing sessions with me seemed fuelled by his fear of loss. I remain unsure if he had reached the stage when the purpose of therapy had been served (Lanyado and Horne 1999). His situation hadn't allowed us to directly address many of his traumatic experiences complete with his anxieties and his humiliation. However, in the playroom I increasingly noticed minute changes in the feelings in the room. There were signs that Kenneth was more able to benefit from positive relationships. The question whether this in future will enable him to better engage with others remains open.

Longer-term reflections on the PBOT process

It was difficult to identify Kenneth's understanding of therapy and yet he looked forward to his sessions and was fully engaged in the process. I was never bored by him; such a feeling might have indicated he or I emotionally shutting down. His emotional state was visible and raw. The fact that he had dared to engage with me was of value. Indeed, in hindsight that was probably the prime purpose of the sessions, one human in meaningful contact with another. I wished that I could have continued to work with him. I say 'work', and it was hard work for us both, as well as *serious play*.

Copley and Forryan (1997, p. 114) advise that 'the feelings about ending often have to be borne by the worker before the client is able to experience any of them himself'. They write (p. 113) of the therapist's anxiety about the adequacy of the child's inner strength at the end of therapy. Kenneth saw himself as strong, but I remained anxious for him. The culture in which he lived was that of poverty, loss, crime and intergenerational trauma. How would he find healthy role models? How would he manage to channel his impulsive and potentially destructive behaviour? I feared he could be drawn into gangs and criminal behaviour, seeking out a position as hero. I feared others would take advantage of him. Would Hailey manage to keep firm boundaries around him? His sense of identity and self-worth were fragile. Kenneth had the capacity to do unforgivable things. Yet we have to remain empathic towards children and pave the way for them to experience enough goodness to give them hope.

There were different things I wished Kenneth could have moved on to after therapy. He had started to abscond from school, sprinting for miles over the countryside causing huge anxiety and expensive use of police time. Surely this could be turned around? Thinking outside of the box I wondered if there might be an adult runner to jog beside him and train him up to run marathons? He longed to drive a car. Could there be an engineer to teach him about the use of tools and how to mend engines?

Sometimes it is difficult to see progress taking place, after all we cannot hope to eradicate the child's suffering. We can only hope it can change to more symbolic forms with less immediate presence and that a new narrative can be formed. In collaboration with high-quality input from Social Work and Education Kenneth did make changes. Small things combined to something significant. Child psychotherapist Monica Lanyado writes about the aftermath of periods of despair in therapy. She suggests watching for moments of 'connection' with a child when there is a sense of 'authentic relatedness'. There were increasing incidents of relatedness with Kenneth, in what he said, did and how he acted.

> However terrible the traumatic experiences may be, if someone is able to listen and hear that cry, there is paradoxically a moment of hope, trust and meeting with another human being, which can become a turning point.
>
> (Lanyado 2018, p. 148)

References list

Bion, W.R. (1962). *Learning from Experience*. Heinemann.

Copley, B., Forryan, B. (1997). *Therapeutic Work with Children and Young People*. Cassell.

Kenrick, J., Lindsey, C., Tollemache, L., eds. (2019). *Creating New Families: Therapeutic Approaches to Fostering, Adoption and Kinship Care*. Routledge, p.105.

Lanyado, M. (1999). Holding and letting go: Some thoughts about the process of ending therapy. *Journal of Child Psychotherapy*, 25 (3), 357–378.

Lanyado, M. (2018). *Transforming Despair to Hope: Reflections on the Psychotherapeutic Process with Severely Neglected and Traumatised Children*. Routledge.

Lanyado, M., Horne, A., eds. (1999). *The Handbook of Child and Adolescent Psychotherapy: Psychoanalytic Approaches*. Routledge.

8

WORKING WITH THE MULTIDISCIPLINARY TEAM

In occupational therapy, as with many clinical professions, there has been an age-old debate around core versus generic roles. Should generic working be embraced when we are part of a multidisciplinary team (MDT)? What are the gains for the service (and the profession) if we perform similar functions to our colleagues in psychology, social work, psychiatry, play therapy or mental health nursing, for instance? Do we risk losing professional identity by blurring those boundaries, becoming 'jacks of all trades' and diluting our skills and models of intervention?

Our experience over many years, is that working within a Child and Adolescent Mental Health Services (CAMHS) service is a truly multidisciplinary experience. Occupational therapists are present in various multidisciplinary teams, providing services across community-based geographical areas, centralised day and inpatient units, and addressing specific issues such as trauma, attention-deficit/hyperactivity disorder and autism, early years support and care for children with prior experiences in the child welfare system. Within these teams, occupational therapists fulfil a core

DOI: 10.4324/9781003642862-9

function, dictated by the needs of the team and the interests and additional training of the individual, including, for example, delivery of cognitive behavioural therapy, anxiety management, social and life skills development or sensory integration. For the writers of this book the core function has been play based assessment and treatment (PBOT), and we shall focus on that modality only.

The occupational therapy generic role will require therapists to take part in initial assessments, often with a colleague from the same team – engaging children and their families when they first arrive in CAMHS. This involves collating a developmental history, discussing the reasons for referral, making a general mental health and risk assessment and arriving at an initial formulation and decision on the way forward. This could be supplying advice or signposting towards appropriate services, accepting the referral into CAMHS and deciding on priority and appropriate intervention or acting where imminent risk is assessed. To achieve a balance between core and generic roles, several issues need to be considered. It is important that there is clarity about what the core role involves, and that it is articulated and agreed with the rest of the team. The service needs in terms of the division of time may require flexibility as pressures change. Questions emerge. Are all clinicians regardless of discipline confident in making a mental health and risk assessment? Is high-quality team function adequately resourced? Can any additional learning required to perform these tasks, be adequately met by co-working with a more experienced member of the team? Might a culture of respect for professional difference and theoretical background be promoted? Are there regular opportunities for sharing knowledge, for case discussions and for clarifying procedures or organisational tasks vital to good team function. Lines of accountability need to be clear – the team lead of an MDT and the occupational therapist's line manager will likely not be the same person.

In our opinion, good practice when working with the complexities of children and their families, requires interdisciplinary working. Meeting with a patient new to CAMHS and their family, can mean a room full of people (e.g., granny, siblings, uncle, neighbour or social worker) who all have useful perspectives to contribute. In years gone by, initial assessment meetings sometimes involved several members of the team, two in the room with the family and the rest behind a viewing screen. This practice no longer takes place to our knowledge, partly because it was recognised as a rather intimidating process for the family, but also as it is very resource heavy. However, it did allow for rich observations of family concerns and dynamics.

During treatment the therapist will often see the child for play based therapy while an MDT colleague is co-working with the parent, perhaps focusing on understanding and managing behaviour and the impact of trauma, attachment and relationship issues or more general support. Appropriate support to parents can sometimes be the most effective intervention. Certainly, the family unit should be seen as a system which may require multi-faceted intervention, rather than treatment of the child in isolation. This requires the range of skills and theoretical frameworks that an MDT provides, promoting the good practice of interdisciplinary working and communication. All clinicians in CAMHS are influenced by the interdisciplinary contributions of other professions. The cross-fertilisation of ideas is a vital component of reflective and effective practice.

Of course, there are challenges to interdisciplinary working. It is likely that the occupational therapist may be the only representative of their profession in any given interdisciplinary situation. A degree of professional isolation is a risk, as is loss of identity. Helping to ameliorate this are such factors as strong occupational therapy management, clear and positive communication and a support and supervision structure. Dynamics of control, divided allegiances or conflict can be played out and perhaps magnified in a large interdisciplinary team. Care is required to keep the best interests of the patient at centre. Dynamics can become split if team members become over-identified with parts of the family system. In our particular CAMHS, in the absence of child psychotherapists, occupational therapists represented the inner world, the unseen experience and voice of the child. This voice is not always easy for adults to hear, even for our multidisciplinary colleagues, and can all too easily be drowned out by the pressing needs of a vulnerable parent or of resource issues.

Working with the professional network

It takes a village to raise a child.

(ancient African proverb, source unknown)

Interdisciplinary working can include colleagues from outside agencies, who are involved within the professional network around the child and family. Indeed, the authors consider that intervention with the child cannot take place without including the wider environment, for example, primary care, community child health services, education, statutory and voluntary agencies involved such as social services, fostering and adoption agencies and family support services to name a few. Often there will be statutory processes in place such as Child Protection, Children's Hearing System (Scotland only), Supervision orders, Looked After and Accommodated Reviews. This interagency approach has been supported by legislation, in particular in Scotland by GIRFEC (Getting it right for every Child 2006), which provides a consistent framework and shared language for promoting, supporting and safeguarding the wellbeing of children and young people. Central to that aim is the need for information sharing, including and supporting families and carers, joint working and decision-making across any agencies involved.

This means that an important and often time-consuming part of our practice is regular communication with the network and attending interagency meetings. Usually initiated by education or social services, the meetings are opportunities for gathering and sharing information and being part of decision-making processes. It is vital to have a current knowledge of local frameworks, guidelines and legislation. For the therapist it is a chance to share their assessment or progress in therapy. Often an important aspect of this is influencing, educating or supporting other agencies towards a greater understanding of the child's presentation, and how they might best provide support. These meetings can be large and intimidating, sometimes tense and conflicted in nature, with difficult decisions having to be made. At best however these processes can be a very positive way of getting everyone involved in an agreed plan of action in which families and children can feel well supported towards the best outcome.

Jonny's (aged 11) behaviour at school had deteriorated dramatically at school. He was described as tired and listless in class, not engaging with learning and had twice struck out at other pupils in the playground. School were aware of his unsettled home life and saw him as a troubled boy, but were concerned they might not manage his more aggressive outbursts. In my sessions with Jonny, he had just begun to play out scenes that seemed directly related to the early traumatic loss of his mum, and I was aware that the current poor health of one of his foster parents was triggering anxiety for him. The teaching assistant who had worked with him in the past was at a loss as to how to engage him. A multi-agency meeting arrived at a decision to support the pupil support assistant to understand Jonny's behaviour through a trauma-focused lens and consider how to schedule activities and time out of the classroom for him. I had some very positive telephone discussions with her over the next couple of weeks and by the time the next meeting was held, things had improved greatly at school, and she was feeling more confident in her role. This outcome reinforced the school's commitment to funding the input.

Child protection

Child protection is a statutory requirement that we are frequently engaged with because of the nature of the children we see. The National Guidance for Child Protection in Scotland (2023) lays out the responsibilities and expectations that every agency and practitioner must follow to safeguard the children they work with. Essentially as therapists we need to be mindful of anything which gives cause for concern about possible harm to a child or young person. That will include concerns about abuse, neglect, exploitation or violence. The same guidance sets out the protocols and processes to be followed. Where a child is deemed to be at risk, the therapist will be required to share information with the other agencies involved, attend interagency meetings and write formal reports.

Sometimes concerns about a child's safety or wellbeing will emerge for the first time during a play session. This could be a comment or action within the metaphor of a play scenario which raises a concern for the therapist, such as a playing out of an act of violence towards a character in the play. These kinds of scenarios happen frequently in children's sessions and are in many ways the 'stuff' of therapy. However, while keeping an open mind on the meaning of the play, the child's current safety must be at the forefront. The violent play could be considered a direct representation of an actual current or past experience. The meaning of the play is rarely clear when it first emerges. For example, Figure 8.1 may represent pride in a family emblem or a wish for protection from outsiders. In the session it would be helpful to consider what kind of comment the child could tolerate within the context of the therapeutic relationship – a reflection staying in the play sequence or something more direct, linking the play with the child's external world. It is important for the therapist to record this in their session notes, discuss within supervision and, if a recurring theme, to discuss this with the child's allocated social worker or duty social worker and, where appropriate, with the parents. Often it is an accumulation of shared concerns over time that builds a clearer understanding of what is going on.

Occasionally a child may make a very clear and definite disclosure about harm within a session. A judgement must be made in the moment as to how much detail of the 'who did what, where and when' the child should be encouraged to share. The therapist's role is not to investigate but to

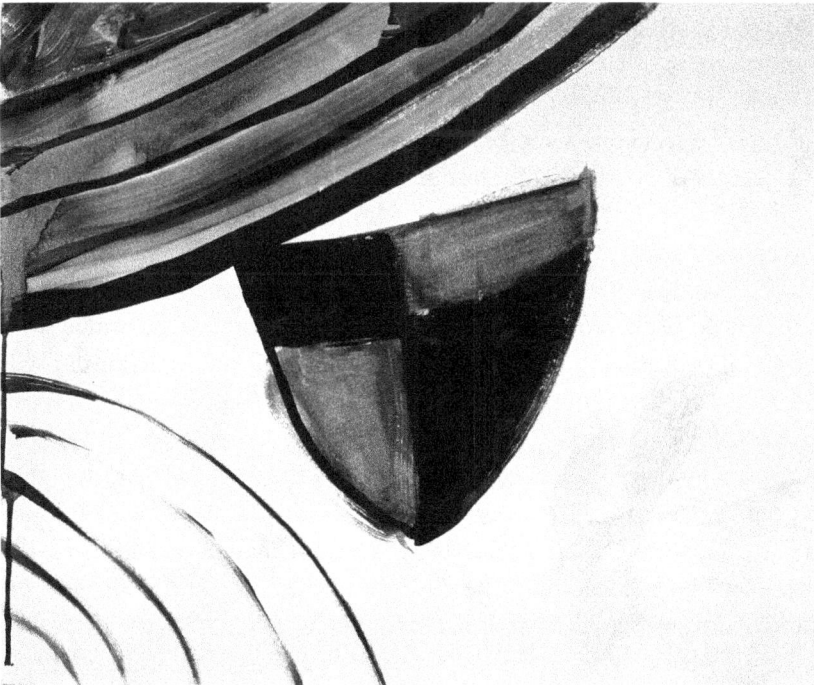

Figure 8.1 'My shield' replica artwork based on a painting by Logan 13 years.

gently ascertain current safety and the approximate timeline of events, using only open and non-leading questions. The child then needs to know what the therapist will do with this information, and to have their courage acknowledged. The disclosure must then be recorded and shared with social services in a timeous manner. Prompt discussion with a supervisor (or experienced member of the team) will be helpful in untangling what has been shared by the child.

Very occasionally the concerns are about a situation which is unsafe and current. Action is then required with a degree of urgency, and sometimes the question arises as to whether the child is safe to leave the session to return home. An understanding of the child's status is necessary (i.e., on the child protection register, supervision order, looked after at home, looked after and accommodated, adopted) and of their living and contact arrangements. The child's allocated social worker or a duty social worker will need to be contacted straight away, and decisions made about the child's immediate care. If an open and positive relationship with the child's social worker has already been formed prior to this event, it will make the sharing of concerns and disclosures an easier process. In official enquiries which have taken place over past decades into the causes of too many tragic cases of child abuse and death, the failure of agencies to share information has consistently been held up as a major contributing factor. The process of good communication cannot be stressed too highly.

In addition to sharing information with our interdisciplinary colleagues, it is important to discuss these events and seek support in supervision. Child protection situations create a good deal of anxiety for even the most experienced of therapists. While the urgent situations are of course stressful for all concerned and will have consequences for the relationship with the child which will need consideration, the situations which are less clear cut should also become a focus in supervision. When scenarios play out in therapy which raise concerns about a harmful experience to the child, but the themes are still emerging over sessions and not yet clearly linked to real events, the therapist's task is to contain that anxiety, within the support from supervision, until there is greater certainty so that sharing with external agencies or family has real meaning.

Formal report writing is part of the process of communication with the professional network, and the issue of confidentiality and honouring the child's communication from within the safe space of the playroom, can be a complex question (more on this in Chapter 5).

Consultation

Consultation with the child's professional network prior to referral, can be used as a one-off discussion forum for all involved to consider whether a referral to CAMHS is appropriate, what alternative support might be more helpful and what advice or support can be offered during a waiting period. Occupational therapists are often involved in these discussions about children with complex backgrounds who may be appropriate for play based therapy.

However, a more in-depth series of consultations for the professional network can be considered when a referral for a care experienced child or late adopted child is received, whether or not the child may also be offered direct therapy. Consultation is not play based or child-led work but often runs parallel with direct intervention with the child. For some children, direct therapy is not indicated at the point of referral. This does not mean that no intervention can be offered, indeed consultation can be the therapy of choice.

Some children may be placed in residential units or in specialist residential schools. Foster care may be short or long term, permanent or temporary. In practice, many short-term placements extend well beyond preferred time scales as suitable resources are in short supply. Children can wait in limbo for years. The question then arises as to how permanent is permanent, how long term is temporary and at what point might it be advisable to use a window of opportunity to engage with a child whilst they are waiting for a permanent placement. Many children are cared for in kinship care with relatives, often grandparents. This brings complex issues of loss and grief to the fore as family members have a close emotional investment in both the children in their care, and in the birthparents from whom the children have been removed – often their own children.

Children in the care system often have a large number of agencies and professionals involved – a team around the child consisting of care staff, school, social work, fostering and adoption agencies, community child health, CAMHS and others. Consultation may involve meeting with the whole system in order to share information and clarify roles and responsi-bilities of those involved.

The type of consultation we will discuss here has a different focus and involves helping those directly involved in offering parenting to the chil-dren in their care. Golding (2004) has outlined the model where

> Consultants draw upon a range of psychological knowledge in response to different problems and issues presented, and in line with the natural styles and abilities of the carers. Frequently, attach-ment theory is used to help understand the behaviour of the child. Equally important is an understanding of how trauma within families impacts on the developing child. Good understanding of child abuse and neglect, the effect of trauma, loss and separation, attachment difficulties and the impact of being fostered is essential prerequisite knowledge for providing consultation to foster carers.
>
> (p. 72)

By understanding how a child's particular traumas and early adversity have affected the subjective experience of the child, carers are more able to tune into the child's inner world. The consultation is about making links between what has happened to the child and their current challenging behaviour, which is often hard to understand. Such consultation meetings should not be too large. In our experience carers appreciate a safe space where they are able to really think about what it is like caring for their child, their concerns about the effects on other children in their care and links with their own previous experiences – what this child brings up for them. The consultation should involve the carers, two CAMHS staff acting as consultants, the child's social worker and the family placement social worker. It is important to have both social workers there, as their priorities may not always tally. For the child's social worker, the priority is to secure and maintain the placement resource and avoid crises or potential break-down, whereas the family placement social worker needs to ensure that the carer(s)' needs are being met. In a world which is often resource rather than needs driven, this can lead to tension in the system. The success of a foster placement can depend on how these two parts communicate and yet, we have found that it is not unusual for the consultation session to be the first time that the two social workers meet. At times, school staff may also be invited.

CASE STUDY OF STAN AGED 11

REFERRAL

Stan was referred due to threatening and at times violent behaviour towards his foster carers, especially his foster mum. She became frightened to be alone in the house with Stan, who developed a fascination with knives. He also did not want to spend time in his bedroom and often wandered the house at night, making the carers worry what he might be up to. Stan continued to have contact with his mother and grandmother twice a year, supervised by the social worker, who had only been involved with Stan for a year. Stan looked forward to these visits, when his mother often came laden with birthday and Christmas presents. The carers tried to help Stan manage these gifts in a positive way but worried about how he would make sense of it all. Stan had lived with his current family for two years and his difficult behaviour had escalated after the placement recently had been made permanent. A referral for consultation was made.

BACKGROUND

Stan was removed from his mother's care at the age of five due to her serious mental illness. She had several periods in hospital due to psychotic episodes, during which time Stan stayed with his maternal grandmother and her partner. This step-grandfather was a heavy drinker and had been known to be a violent man. When Stan was five years old there was a house fire in his mother's house. Although no one was seriously hurt, this was catalyst for Stan being removed from his mother's care. Her condition remained unstable, and it was considered that she was not able to offer him the care he needed. He was initially placed with his grandmother and her partner, who eventually applied for a kinship care order to look after him permanently. However, she failed the assessment for this, and Stan was moved to a single female carer for a year, prior to his placement with his current specialist carers.

ISSUES FOR CONSULTATION

- Careful examining of health and social work files, building up as clear a picture of Stan's life as possible.

- A timeline of significant events in Stan's life, from his perspective. Speculation of how he might have experienced these events. Alternatively, creating a genogram of Stan's family and relationships may have been created. Such visual representations of a child's life can be enlightening.
- A space for carers to be open about their concerns for Stan, for themselves and for their wider family – they had grandchildren who visited.
- A space for the social workers to voice their concerns. Especially the family placement social worker was very much in touch with the distress of the carers and whether this placement could continue.

By focusing on the first two points, it became clear that the other concerns were also beginning to be addressed.

The consultants spent a morning in preparation for the consultation, studying health and social work files. It was not possible to contact mother's psychiatrist to find out about the exact nature of her psychosis. However, they noted her frequent delusional and paranoid outbursts and speculated what this may have been like for a young child to witness and manage. Equally they found out that the house fire had involved Stan being blocked in his room by the fire and only rescued by the emergency services. He was briefly admitted to hospital with smoke inhalation.

The session itself focused on creating a timeline, and these above issues were highlighted as significant to the situation with Stan now. The social worker seemed surprised to hear about the fire at all, and the carers had also not been aware of the severity of the incident. Where children's lives are characterised by many changes in placements and staff, it is unfortunately not unusual for facts to be lost altogether or the significance of them minimised. The consultation offered a chance for the consultees to tune into Stan's traumatised and fearful early life. The carers were able to speculate as to the link between Stan's unexpressed and confused feelings towards his mother and his wariness and anger at his current foster mother. Could the two be connected? Was Stan harbouring hopes of being reunited with his mother in his late teens? Did he worry about her wellbeing? Stan's fear of spending time in his bedroom at night suddenly began to make sense. Was his traumatisation by the fire compounded by the fact that in his mind it had also led to the separation from his mother?

Stan's carers expressed worry and exasperation about Stan, but they also began to feel real empathy and curiosity as to how he could be helped. Stan had a 'life-story book', detailing his early life. But this was very general, speaking only about the fact that his mother was 'poorly and not able to care for him'. The fire was not mentioned. The carers understood that he needed a more nuanced and truthful explanation about his life to date. The social worker expressed a willingness to meet with Stan to try and talk with him and think with him about his life, using drawing. The foster mother expressed a desire to join these meetings if appropriate.

We agreed to meet again in three months' time to review the situation. One of the consultants circulated a note detailing the concerns, the discussion and the outcome of the consultation to all concerned.

Almost every consultation with carers includes a consideration about contact with birthparents or other family members. Loxtercamp (2009) in his paper *Contact and truth: The unfolding predicament in adoption and fostering* has questioned the assumption that contact that appears to be going well will naturally meet the child's need for a sense of belonging with their origins. The meaning of contact needs considered. What are children told about their early experiences? As in the case of Stan and his carers, important information is often lost, withheld or glossed over by professionals. His life-story book did not represent his true experiences and therefore could not help him form a realistic picture of his family. He was looking forward to seeing his mother who generously would bring him presents. Without knowing the full facts, having been permanently removed from her may not have made much sense to him. The idea that he wants to return to live with her in the future may well grow. It was therefore not surprising that it was the foster mother who was at the receiving end of all his angry and confused feelings. The loss that Stan had endured was unalterable. Loxtercamp states that

What a child needs most of all is help to come to terms with that loss and its causes, help to manage knowing and understanding the harrowing explanation that will explain (with greater sophistication as the child matures) why he had to be removed permanently from the birth

> family. Without this knowledge, it is likely that the child will come to be injuriously convinced, for example, that he is blameworthy because he wasn't good enough for his birthparents, or that he is being prevented from returning to his parent for no good reason.
>
> (p. 434)

This is work which needs undertaken with Stan. In his case he will also need some understanding of his mother's illness, to be absolved from any guilt that he as a young child was not able to look after her and acknowledgement of his fear that he may be prone to a mental illness himself.

Working with the family

Key to good outcomes for children is the involvement of their parents. All interventions with children need to include the families, whether it be to achieve a complete assessment, to liaise with family through the ups and downs of therapy or to provide parallel work with the parents themselves.

During a series of play based sessions, it is helpful if parents know they can contact the therapist about the impact sessions may be having on their child, or major issues or changes arising for them at home or at school. However, it is important that those conversations do not take place with the child present at the beginning or endings of sessions. Play based sessions can be an anxious time for parents, wondering how children will manage and what they will talk about with the therapist. It is useful to let parents know that they will receive feedback at the end of the assessment period or the next review, but they can make contact at other times if necessary. We discuss how to share the outcome from an assessment with the family in Chapter 5.

During ongoing play based work, reviewing the child's sessions with parents needs to happen regularly. A decision should be made about whether it is helpful for the child to be present for the whole or part of that discussion, which will depend on the age and stage of the child, the child's wishes, what is to be shared from their sessions or any other agenda for the discussion. It may be helpful to have colleagues from the professional network present also. It is good practice to follow up review meetings with a written summary of what was discussed.

Play based therapy often involves parallel work with parents by an MDT colleague. Several interventions can be appropriate

- psychoeducation around the impact of trauma on brain development
- considering their child's behaviour through a trauma-focused lens and how best to manage those behaviours
- helping their child build skills for emotional and stress regulation, which may involve the parent considering their own self-management
- consideration of relationships and dynamics within the family and the parent's attachment to the child
- attachment-focused parenting encouraging the parent's capacity for reflection on the child's internal experience, for thinking about the meaning of a behaviour before responding to it
- help with specific issues such as poor sleep, eating issues and social skills.

It is worth repeating that sometimes the most effective intervention is not with the child, but with the parent only. This could be short-term support for the parent's own issues until an appropriate service can be accessed elsewhere. It may be that it is not the right time for the child to be seen, or that foundation skills need to be developed before PBOT can be effective. It would then be appropriate to work on some of the above issues with the parents or carers alone. Chloe's 'Assessment review and treatment plan' in Chapter 5, gives a summary of how individual assessment sessions were shared with the system around her and resulted in further work with the carers rather than Chloe alone.

Reference list

Golding, K. (2004). Providing specialist psychological support to foster carers: A consultation model. *Child and Adolescent Mental Health*, 9 (2), 71–76.

'It takes a village to raise a child' (ancient African proverb, source unknown).

Loxtercamp, L. (2009). Contact and truth: The unfolding predicament in adoption and fostering. *Clinical Child Psychology and Psychiatry*, 14, 423–434.

Scottish Government. (2006). *Getting It Right for Every Child, Implementation Plan*. Scottish Government.

Scottish Government. (2023). *National Guidance for Child Protection in Scotland 2021 – Updated 2023*. Scottish Government Publications.

9

SUPERVISION AND SUPPORT

Therapists cannot practice without supervision. Supervision has been described as 'extra-vision' (Inskipp and Proctor 1988). It is an inter-relational space (Casement 2002), where supervisee and supervisor are learning together from experience. The process is underpinned by estab-lished theoretical understanding and emerging ideas. Two minds come together to think about clinical case material in a regular, confidential, uninterrupted and safe space. Here ideas can be explored and played with. How can we understand particular ways of relating, or find meaning in play and activity that may seem confusing? Practical approaches can be worked out about what to say to the child, how to move, and how to man-age time and equipment.

The setting is akin to Winnicott's holding environment (1971) and Bion's containing space (1962). McMahon (2014) considers a cornerstone of supervision being the development of a relationship that can support both personal and professional growth. The supervisor can offer knowledge and experience with humility, so that both vulnerability and competence in

DOI: 10.4324/9781003642862-10

the therapist are valued. There are times when a supervisor may need to challenge a supervisee in relation to some aspects of the work. Cutcliffe and Mcfeely (2001) believe that trust and safety balanced with challenge is necessary for supervision to be effective, honest and supportive.

Clinical supervision is different from line management. In the case of occupational therapists, the line manager will usually be an occupational therapist, whereas a supervisor can come from a variety of professional backgrounds with whom the therapist can find a suitable 'fit'. Supervision may be provided either inhouse or bought in externally. It can be face to face or online. Whereas online therapy with young children poses many challenges, supervision lends itself more easily to the use of a screen. This brings many benefits in terms of overcoming problems of distance and time-consuming travel, thereby increasing the likelihood of finding suitable supervisors. If possible, it is helpful to have at least one initial face to face meeting for supervisee and supervisor to experience sharing a physical space together as they build up mutual trust.

The contract between supervisor and supervisee varies in how formally it is drawn up. Whatever the format, it is helpful to think together about the parameters of the work so that expectations can be clear on both sides. A yearly review of the supervisory relationship can be valuable to make sure that unmet needs can be explored, rather than supervisees running the risk of adapting silently to the style of the supervisor (McMahon 2022).

A central aspect of supervision is allowing the supervisee a space to reflect on and explore their own feelings evoked by the therapy. Therapists are frequently required to contain and manage highly distressing material. One's own emotional responses to the child can, through projective identification (see Chapter 6), give important clues as to what is going on for the child. However, therapists need to consider carefully what feelings belong where and when personal feelings are triggered in the countertransference (see Chapter 6). If it is felt that such feelings become overwhelming and get in the way of therapeutic practice, the supervisor may encourage the supervisee to seek additional help in a personal capacity. Clinical supervision will be enhanced by self-supervision in the form of session notes made in a reflective way.

Discussing dilemmas informally with colleagues can be an important support mechanism to complement more formal supervision. Therapists also have a responsibility to keep up to date with current practice developments and literature through their own professional inquiry. These support mechanisms are time consuming and can be expensive; however, it is well acknowledged that they increase effectiveness, reduce stress and burnout and improve morale (Evans 2001). They can also provide protection against therapists experiencing symptoms of secondary trauma. By this we refer to individuals experiencing traumatisation as a result of ongoing exposure to traumatic events in others. Therapists and other staff working with children with experiences of abuse are particularly vulnerable to this.

Good supervision allows for thinking about both internal and external aspects of the therapy. We start by considering the internal mindset of the therapist. In her seminal paper 'On creating a psychotherapeutic space' (1991), Monica Lanyado points to the therapist's mind needing to be genuinely free of anything that will dilute the intensity of attentiveness to the child. The therapist needs to be able to manage their own anxiety and hold intense emotional pain and shocking details of trauma communicated through play and words.

Below are three excerpts of play with Jane aged 5, which illustrate the dovetailing of the child's feelings with those of the therapist.

Jane 5 yrs (also discussed in chapter 4) had attended weekly sessions for three months. She usually settled quickly into the playroom to paint and play and would often take off her socks and shoes, thus claiming her space. On this occasion she seemed agitated. She threw toys around, ran in and out of the room and insisted on using the real phone instead of the toy phone to dial 999.

When it was time to finish, I told Jane she had 5 minutes left. She ran out of the room and then back in. In just a few seconds she had thrown dry sand all around the playroom. I tried to help her put on her socks and shoes. She threw them away and became more emotionally heightened. I felt confused and aware of how like a toddler she could be. She threw sand at me and shouted, 'I hate you!' A colleague heard her shouts and entered the room. Immediately Jane calmed down and we accompanied her back to her foster carers.

We need to think before we can understand. This situation did not leave space for thinking. Balancing the therapist's own anxiety with any understanding of the child's feelings and communications proved difficult. As a result, opportunities were missed to bring some reciprocity into the session.

Exploration in supervision can help connect thoughts, feelings and ideas. The role of supervision is to offer a space where the therapist can process this material. This includes thinking about how the change in Jane's behaviour can be understood and whether her communication can be put into context. Maintaining an observational stance (see Chapter 6) in such a difficult session gives rise to many questions. The therapist's own feelings during this session were those of helplessness and confusion. Those may have mirrored how Jane had felt during traumatic events in her life. Can the child be given a sense of the therapist's ability to emotionally tolerate and think about such communications without fear that they might be acted on in unhelpful ways? Can therapy continue safely? Thinking through possible responses to Jane was vital in order to ensure that she would not feel that she had destroyed the relationship between herself and the therapist. In supervision the therapist can play with questions of 'what if', almost as a rehearsal for next similar time. In Jane's session, had the therapist become more aware of the early signs of Jane's heightening emotional state, it might have been possible to find a way of naming her feelings. The therapist and the supervisor also considered practical ways to help Jane manage transitions, in particular into the therapy room and out of the room in order to make her sessions as safe as possible.

Moving from the space of the therapy room, we need to consider what Lanyado calls an 'external therapeutic space' (1991). This includes parents, teachers, social workers and the multidisciplinary team. In Jane's case, the supervisor drew attention to the need for effective support for the foster carers within the wider system, and for this support to be linked to the themes which Jane brought to her sessions. At the very least Jane's foster carers needed to feel looked after and that their experience of secondary trauma in relation to Jane was understood. Supervision provides a space to think carefully about whether there is sufficient support for play based occupational therapy in the frequently complex networks which surround the child.

Staying with Jane, the example below is a tragic reflection of a professional system under strain. The external therapeutic space was not sufficiently robust to manage an unexpected crisis in the foster family. A lack of effective communication in the network led to a sudden breakdown in placement and insufficient preparation for the new carers. During this time the therapist was in need of extra supervision, such was the pain in this rupture. Particularly because Jane was so young she seemed to provoke strong maternal, protective feelings in the therapist. It is not unusual for therapists to grasp at straws and wish to take the child home with them. Instead of this unrealistic scenario Jane was placed in temporary foster care.

Jane had attended weekly sessions for six months. In parallel her long-term foster carers had been offered support to better understand and manage Jane's challenging behaviour. Unfortunately, however, a sudden serious illness in the carers' extended family meant that they no longer felt able to continue to care for little Jane safely. The placement ended abruptly and she was moved into temporary foster care. These new carers, knowing little of the ongoing therapeutic work, had been told to bring Jane to her appointment.

In the waiting room, in front of Jane the carers asked the therapist what the purpose of the appointment was. There had been no opportunity for anyone to explain this to them. In that moment something of Jane's experience was transferred to the therapist. The work which Jane and her previous carers had undertaken felt diminished. This was undermining of the therapeutic process and of Jane's ability to express herself and tell her own story. The therapist felt bewildered and angry and struggled to explain the purpose of the appointment, given the public space of the waiting room and the time pressure. Jane's session below reflects the impact of the sudden external changes in her life. She expressed clearly that something was very wrong.

Jane immediately took my hand and led the way from the waiting room to the playroom. I told her that I knew she had moved to live with different people and was having to say goodbye to the carers she and I knew so well. She agreed but spoke no more of them.

As usual she took off her socks and shoes. She then climbed into the sand tray. She pulled up one leg of her trousers explaining that she had broken her leg and that it was 'in one hundred pieces'. She told me to be a doctor and pour sand over her leg. I did so, quietly and gently for some time. She was still and watched the sand flow over her leg.

She told me that the sand is blood. She asked me to inject her leg to get the blood into her leg and make it better. I enacted this. After a while she sighed and said, 'we can't make the blood go in, it's just still coming out.'

I was struggling with my own sadness for this little girl and just said, 'it is so hard for us to stop the hurt.'

Jane told me to put her to bed and as she lay on the sand, she directed me to spread a sheet over her and tuck it around her. I did so. She asked me to put a plaster on as she wanted us to fix her leg. With sadness she realised how impossible this was and said, 'it cannot fix.'

I acknowledged that the leg was still sore, and she was sad. She moved her leg towards me showing me that it remained broken.

Clinical supervision had allowed for exploration of the sadness and helplessness felt by the therapist as a way in to understanding how things were for Jane, who in fact showed a remarkable ability to be in touch with her deep sadness. One could say she was able to stay in what Melanie Klein (Segal 1988) called the depressive position (see Chapter 6). The therapist was able to stay with Jane's pain, helping her to feel understood rather than try to make better what could not be changed. Supervision helped contain the therapist's sorrow, enabling her to connect to other (personal) losses she had experienced. It helped her to include the richness of those experiences into the therapy room and not shy away from those feelings.

Bringing this chapter to an end leaves us with important questions to consider. Do the organisations within which we practise have the capacity to support such work through the right job plans, supervision structure and a culture of peer support and reflective practice? The requirements for throughput and meeting of targets in increasingly overstretched CAMHS departments need balanced by a climate where curious inquiry and awareness of unconscious processes can also be supported and encouraged (Hoxter 1983).

Below is an example of a multidisciplinary support structure for individual play based therapy. Occupational therapists in CAMHS coordinated a monthly multidisciplinary reflective practice group, led by an external facilitator, offering peer support through work discussion and the reading of relevant theoretical and practice papers. Those of any professional background were welcome. The thinking shared within the group was from a psychodynamic perspective. This was a well-attended and vibrant group, and the benefits are illustrated by the following statements given by group members as evaluation.

The reading has brought up cases from my own experience - this has at times been an emotional experience. This is also the case with listening to other people's cases. The experience of the group is further enriched by the reading material.

It is helpful to link theory and practice. It's a lifeline for my work to be able to come here and top myself up. If I did not have this group, I could not do the play based work.

I often discuss the papers with others in my team and elsewhere. I build up my own personal library of helpful papers, to be used as and when.

The group provides a depth of discussion that you don't get at team away days.

This group gives value to the therapeutic relationship and not just a quick fix - so necessary in work with complex trauma.

Reference list

Bion, W.R. (1962a). *Learning from Experience.* Heinemann.

Casement, B. (2002). *Learning from Our Mistakes: Beyond Dogma in Psychoanalysis and Psychotherapy.* Brunner Routledge.

Cutcliffe, J., Mcfeely, S. (2001). Practice nurses and their 'lived experience' of supervision. *British Journal of Nursing,* 10 (5), 312–314 and 316–323.

Evans, S. (2001). Keeping safe: Supervision and support. Ch 14. In Lougher L. ed. *Occupational Therapy for Child and Adolescent Mental Health.* Churchill Livingstone, pp. 221–238.

Hoxter, S. (1983). Feelings aroused in working with severely deprived children. Ch 15. In Boston, M., Szur, R. eds. *Psychotherapy with Severely Deprived Children*. Karnac, pp. 125–132.

Inskipp, F., Proctor, B. (1988). Skills for supervising and being supervised. Cited in Lougher, L., ed. (2001). *Occupational Therapy in Child and Adolescent Mental Health*. Churchill Livingstone, p. 222.

Lanyado, M. (1991). On creating a psychotherapeutic space. *Journal of Social Work Practice*, 5 (1), 31–40.

McMahon, A. (2014). Four guiding principles for the supervisory relationship. In *Reflective Practice: International and Multidisciplinary Perspectives*, 15 (3), 333–346.

McMahon, A. (2022). *Vulnerability and Humility in Supervision Relationships*. Training Notes, Relationship Scotland Inhouse Training October 2022.

Segal, H. (1988). *Introduction to the Work of Melanie Klein*. Karnac.

Winnicott, D.W. (1971). *Playing and Reality*. Routledge.

FINAL THOUGHTS

We began this writing project as a small group of therapists who were concerned that a valuable way of working with children who had experienced complex trauma, was in danger of becoming overlooked and under-resourced amidst the escalating demands on Child and Adolescent Mental Health Services. Our hope was to inspire new therapists, and support those already using child-led play as a way of working. We also hoped to encourage workers within children's services to feel comfortable and validated in the use of play as a means of communicating with children.

There is convincing evidence that the life trajectory of traumatised children into adulthood is not a positive one. Statistics relating to difficulties within education, employment, finances, housing, physical and mental health, addiction and prison, often track back to trauma in childhood. Surely resourcing early and effective intervention to alter that trajectory would benefit children, families and society itself. Child-led therapy may not be a quick fix, but for some children it is the only way of engaging.

There is no doubt that distilling the life stories of these children and their therapy, has been an opportunity for reflection on our own therapeutic practice. In bringing these life stories together we were reminded what grim lives some children experience, and yet behind each story was a real relationship within the playroom, where connection, laughter and

DOI: 10.4324/9781003642862-11

discovery were also experienced. We applaud the courage and tenacity of the children and families we have worked with along their journey to change.

We hold these children in mind long after we bid them farewell.

Carrie

It was her last session, after many months of therapy, many ups and downs, painful and challenging moments. In the last few minutes, she rummaged about in the cupboard and found the tattered baby, the playmobile girl with the red skirt and the adult female figure (all familiar characters in her play). She placed them carefully in the front row of the toy bus. They were on a journey - 'to Mars' - she added, as the bus careered around the floor, navigating furniture, bumps of the carpet, discarded toys and wet patches. When I wondered aloud if it felt like we had been on a long and difficult journey, 'to Mars and back' she said, 'it's just as well I've learned how to drive'.

INDEX

Note: *Italic* page numbers refer to figures.

abandonment 8, 34, 94
abuse 4, 5, 11, 12; emotional 18–19; physical 15–17; sexual 13–15; types of 13–19
accountability 111
adverse childhood experiences (ACES) 12, 37
aggression 96, 97, 103
Ainsworth, A.D.S. 20, 83
Anda, R.F. 12
The Anna Freud Centre 81
anxiety 27, 34, 52, 72, 116; extreme 28; overwhelming 12
art activities 42; materials 41
assessments 2, 3, 7, 38, 59–65, 75, 80, 122; activities 61–65; my family 61–62, *62*; my island 62–63; review and treatment plan 72–73; three wishes 63–65, *64*
attachment 35, 42, 59, 79; disruptions 11; relationships 11, 36, 76; security 23, 83; styles 67, 79, 83; theory 83, 118

attention deficit hyperactivity disorder (ADHD) 28, 30, 105
autism 26, 28–30, 110
Axline, V.M. 89, 90

Bick, E. 76
Bion, W.R. 60, 82–84, 98, 124
Blunden, P. 3
Boswell, S. 87
Boulton, S. 18
boundaries 33, 87; difficulties 45; ethical 75; professional 75; psychological 19
Bowlby, J. 83
brain development 5, 79, 123
Brooks, R. 3
BUSS model 30

care experienced children 58, 61, 117
Carrie 1, 133
Casement, B. 124
Child Abuse Public Inquiries 15
child psychotherapy 36, 76, 87, 109, 112

Child and Adolescent Mental Health Services (CAMHS) 2–4, 8, 9, 22, 25, 26, 38–40, 56, 59, 67, 76, 95, 100, 110–112, 117, 130

child-led 3, 61, 87, 90, 117; engagement 58; play 2, 56, 66, 81, 132; sessions 73; therapy 67, 132

child protection 8, 113–117; definition of 114; issues 66; professionals 49; services 25

child refugees 5, 22–24

child's natural occupation 3, 6, 32–40

Child Trauma Academy 80

Chloe 68–72

clinical observation 75

clinical supervision 9, 125, 129

communication 2, 4, 6, 9, 32–40, 47, 60, 83; formal report writing 116–117; forms of 83–84; interagency 65; language as 34; reciprocal 96

complex post-traumatic stress disorder (C-PTSD) 11

complex trauma 2–5, 8, 10–21, 28, 58, 59, 80, 86, 87, 94; definition of 5, 11; domestic violence 15–17; emotional abuse 18–19; harmful/ inappropriate sexual behaviour 19–20; indication of 37; mental health difficulties 17–18; neglect 13; neurodivergence 28, 29; parental addiction 17–18; physical abuse 15–17; sense of self and on identity 12–20; sexual abuse 13–15

confidentiality 42, 49, 50, 66, 93, 116

consultation 100, 117–122; care system 117–118; case study 119–121; issues for 119–121; multidisciplinary 8; type of 118

Contact and Truth: The Unfolding predicament in adoption and fostering (Loxtercamp) 121

contain: container/contained 98; containing function 82; containment 89, 98

coping strategies 12, 85

Copley, B. 34, 37, 98, 108

countertransference 7, 76, 85, 107

cross-fertilisation of ideas 8, 112

Cudmore, L. 87

cultural experience 35

Cutcliffe, J. 125

Daws, D. 33

defence mechanisms 49, 85–86

depressive position 78, 82, 129

de Rementeria, A. 33

development/developmental: deficits 11; delays 2, 68; difficulties 11; history 59, 65, 66, 111; stages 6, 54; trauma 11, 30, 68

Diagnostic and Statistical Manual of Mental Disorders (DSM-5) 26

Dibs in Search of Self (Axline) 90

domestic violence 4, 11, 15–17

Evans, S. 126

Emanuel, L. 87

emotion/emotional 16, 34, 37, 46, 49; abuse 18–19; closeness 14; dysregulation 11; exploration 6; growth 8; neglect 18; regulation 2, 73; unavailability 19

ending therapy 8, 94

evidence-based practice 38

external therapeutic space 87, 127, 128

extra-vision 124

families 11, 18, 37; child refugees 22–23; consultation 122–123; neglectful 13; systemic 86–87, 111–112;

feedback 66, 67, 72

Felliti, V.J. 12

Filial Therapy 38

financial insecurity 79

foetal alcohol syndrome 65

formulation 28, 59, 64, 66, 79, 87, 111

Forryan, B. 34, 37, 98, 108
foster care 117, 128
freeze reaction 87
Freud, A. 81
Freud, S. 81
Froebel, F. 32

gaming online 24
gender dysphoria 6, 26–28
Gibertoni, C.de S. 7, 39, 88, 89
GIRFEC (Getting it Right for Every
    Child), Scottish Government 113
Glaser, D. 19
Golding, K. 118
'good enough mother' 84
grief 78, 117
guilt 17, 122

harm 15, 19–20, 114; disclosure of 115;
    self-2, 10, 24, 26–28
harmful sexual behaviours 19–20
Heimann, P. 85
Herman, J.L. 11
Hindle, D. 18
Horne, A. 26, 35, 61, 94, 105
Hoxter, S. 41
Hunter, M. 14
hyper-alert 17, 18
hyper-arousal 13, 80
hypervigilant 16

identity 12–20, 27
illustrations 5, 61–65; 'a beautiful
    rainbow' 51; 'a broken car' 30;
    'family' 69; 'me and my foster
    mum' 12; 'me being made to
    eat something horrible' 16; 'my
    brain' 105; 'my dance' 53; 'my
    family' 62; 'my sad painting'
    53; 'my shield' 115; 'my three
    wishes' 64; 'this is me' 47; 'the
    turtle' 97; 'who is at home?' 50;
    'zig zags' 81
imagination 34, 36

inappropriate sexual behaviour
    19–20, 49
Ingram, G. 85
inner world 8, 63, 82, 83, 112, 118
Inskipp, F. 124
individuality 19
individual therapy 42, 75, 83
intellectual disability 45, 47, 47, 105
interagency communication 65
interdisciplinary working 111–113
internalisation 84
International Classificatory System of
    Diseases (ICD-11) 11
internet 24–26; forums 25;
    monitoring 24; pornography 24
interventions 3, 4, 28, 58, 80, 123
introjection 83
isolation 12; loneliness and 46; social
    26, 79

Jeffrey, L.I.H. 3
Jennifer 54–55
Jung, C. 35

Kenneth 100–108
Kenrick, J. 99
kinship care 117
Klein, M. 82, 84, 129

language of play 3, 34
Lanyado, M. 15, 61, 87, 94, 105, 109,
    126, 127
Lemma, A. 26, 27
letters, therapeutic use of 54–55
Lloyd, S. 30
lockdown 54, 56
loneliness 34, 46
loving environment 79
Loxtercamp, L. 121
loyalty 14, 17

Maté, D. 10
Maté, G. 10
Mcfeely, S. 125

McMahon, A. 124, 125
McNeish, D. 19
Melzak, S. 23
MDT *see* multidisciplinary team
    (MDT)
medical conditions 65
mental health 19; difficulties 17–18;
    disorders 58; parental 4, 11;
    services 4; support 30
mirroring 43
motivation to play 33, 39
MOVI *see* Vivaio model of
    occupational therapy (MOVI)
multidisciplinary team (MDT) 8, 59,
    110–123; child protection 114–117;
    consultation 117–122; working
    with family 122–123; working with
    professional network 112–114
Music, G. 13, 29, 36, 86

National Guidance for Child
    Protection in Scotland (2023)
    18–19, 114
neglect 4, 5, 13, 36; detrimental
    impact of 80
neurodivergence 6, 28–30, 30
neuroscience 75, 80–81, 81
Neurosequential Model of
    Therapeutics (2006) 80
Nicholls, L. 88

Objects Relations Theory 82
observational skills 4, 75, 76, 85
observational stance 7, 76–78, 127
occupational therapy 3–6, 39–40, 76,
    110, 111
*Occupational Therapy for Child and
    Adolescent Mental Health* 85
omnipotence 47, 104
online child abuse 25
organisation 4, 9, 30, 80, 87, 129;
    organisational 111

pandemic 54
parallel play 34
paranoid-schizoid position 82
parental addiction 17–18, 65
parental mental health 4, 11
Parent Infant Psychotherapy 38
parenting 37, 67, 84, 118
PBOT *see* play based occupational
    therapy (PBOT)
peer relationships 28
Perry, B.D. 79, 80
person-centred therapy 89–91
phone calls, therapeutic use of 55–56
physical: abuse 15–17, *16*; assault 14;
    closeness 14; rumbustiousness 37;
    skills 35
Piergrossi, J.C. 7, 88, 89
planning 7, 67–72
play 1–3, 13; children not be able
    to 36–37; as child's natural
    occupation 3, 6, 32–40; as
    communication 6, 32–40; as a
    continuum 33–35; occupational
    therapy and 39–40; purpose of
    35; sense of agency 3; serious 108;
    violent 114
play as therapy 4, 28;
    multidisciplinary team 123;
    principles of 90–91
play based occupational therapy
    (PBOT) 7, 58, 59, 74–91; cases
    95–108; clinical observation 75;
    definition of 3; early experiences,
    importance of 79; longer-term
    reflections 108–109; MOVI
    model of occupational therapy
    87–89; neuroscience 80–81,
    81; person-centred therapy
    and 89–91; psychoanalytic
    thinking, influence of 81–83;
    psychodynamic observational
    stance 76–78; psychodynamic

theories 83–86; systemic understanding 86–87; theories informing 75, 76
playing: adults' attitudes to 37–39; childhood 35;toddlers 34
Playing and Reality (Winnicott) 39
playroom 6–7, 41–57, 66, 117; child orientation 44–45; child's anxiety 52, 53; child's confidentiality 49, 50; child's entry 43; child's feelings 46; child's interaction 46–48, 47; child's pace 51, 51–52; helpful response 50–51;manage boundary difficulties 45; materials, use 45–46; pointless activity 52; therapists learn from the child 44
pornography 24
post-traumatic stress disorder (PTSD) 23
poverty 11, 79
pretend play 34
Proctor, B. 124
projection 84
projective identification 46, 84
Psychanalytic Thinking in Occupational Therapy (Piergrossi & Gibertoni) 88
psychoanalysis 4, 7
psychoanalytic thinking 81–83
psychodynamic observational stance 76–78
psychodynamic theories 83–86; countertransference 85; defence mechanisms 85–86; projection 84; projective identification 84; transference 84–85
psychoeducation 123
psychotherapy 39

rationalisation 85
Reade, S. 2
reciprocal interactions 33

recommendations 15, 59, 66, 67
referrals 2, 4, 22, 26, 59, 117, 119
reflection 4, 43, 48, 69–72, 76, 78, 97–99, 101–105, 107–108, 115, 123, 128, 132; reflective practice 4, 9, 129, 130
report writing 116, 117
Respark (Music) 13
review 7, 65–67
risk assessment 111
Rodgers, C. 89
role play 96
Rory 95–99

Scottish Government x–xi
Scott, S. 19
secondary trauma 126, 127
Seigal, D.J. 36
self: harm 10, 27; portrait 47; realisation 35; supervision 125
sense of belonging 121
sense of self 12–20, 33, 35
separation 34, 35, 42, 44
sexual abuse 13–15, 19
shame 14, 17
Sinason, V. 34
social: isolation 26, 79; media 24, 35; play 34; services 116; worker 49, 72, 100, 104, 115, 116, 118–121
societal issues 11
socio-political issues 8
Stan 119–121
Steiner, D. 32
stress hormones 80
stress regulation pathways 80
Stubley, J. 11
substance misuse 4, 11
supervision 9, 43, 76, 78, 115; clinical 9, 125, 129; definition of 124; exploration 127; internet 24; role of 127; and support 9, 124–130
systemic theory 86

temporary playroom 42
theory base 74
therapeutic process 8, 93–109
Theraplay 38
toys 41–42
toxic hormones 80
transference 83–85; *see also*
    countertransference
transitioning 27
trauma 10; child refugees and 22–24;
    chronic neglect and 13; definitions
    of 11; detrimental impact of
    80; developmental 11, 30, 68;
    disturbance and 87; domestic
    violence 16; focused 67, 80, 90,
    114, 123; gender dysphoria and
    26–28; informed 90; internet
    and 24–26; neurodivergence
    and 28–30, *30*; vulnerabilities
    to 5–6, 22–30; *see also* complex
    trauma

traumatic events 4, 11, 126
trust 8, 10, 13, 17, 125

use dependent brain 80

Van der Kolk, B.A. 11
Vetere, A. 87
video calls, therapeutic use of 56–57
violence 1, 36, 61, 104; domestic 4,
    11, 15–17; upheaval and 23
Vivaio model of occupational therapy
    (MOVI) 7, 39, 76, 87–89
vulnerabilities 5–6, 17, 19, 22–30, 47,
    124

Waddell, M. 35
Winnicott, D.W. 13, 33, 35, 39, 82, 85,
    124
without memory or desire 60, 82

Zeedyk, S. 79, 80

For Product Safety Concerns and Information please contact our EU
representative GPSR@taylorandfrancis.com
Taylor & Francis Verlag GmbH, Kaufingerstraße 24, 80331 München, Germany

www.ingramcontent.com/pod-product-compliance
Lightning Source LLC
Chambersburg PA
CBHW070345270326
41926CB00017B/4002

9 7 8 1 0 4 1 0 7 9 2 2 4